F

THE AMERICAN YOGA ASSOCIATION
BEGINNER'S MANUAL

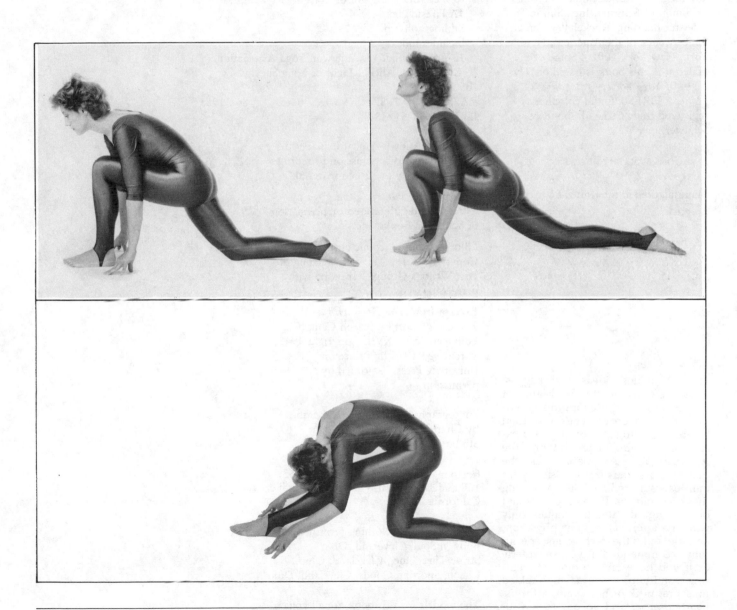

ALICE CHRISTENSEN

A FIRESIDE BOOK • PUBLISHED BY SIMON & SCHUSTER, INC. • NEW YORK

CARTOONS BY KATHY DETZER

Manufactured in the United States of America

10 9 8 7 6 5 4 3 2 1

The techniques, ideas and suggestions presented in this book are not intended to substitute for proper medical advice. Consult your physician before beginning this or any new exercise program. The author, the American Yoga Association, and the publisher assume no responsibility for injuries suffered while practicing these techniques. If you are pregnant or nursing, do the techniques only with the approval of your physician, and do only the techniques specifically recommended. If you are elderly or if you have any chronic or recurring conditions such as high blood pressure, neck or back pain, arthritis, heart disease, and so on, seek your physician's advice about which techniques you should avoid.

Library of Congress Cataloging-in-Publication Data

Christensen, Alice.
    The American Yoga Association beginner's manual.

    Rev. ed. of: The Light of Yoga Society. 1974, c1972.
    "A Fireside book."
    Bibliography: p.
    Includes index.
    1. Yoga, Hatha.   I. American Yoga Association.
II. Christensen, Alice.   Light of Yoga Society.
III. Title.
RA781.7.C5   1987   613.7'046   86-31951
ISBN: 0-671-61935-7

Grateful acknowledgment is made to the following for permission to reprint from previously published material:

Excerpt from *Patanjali and Yoga* by Mircea Eliade. Reprinted by permission of Schocken Books, Inc.

"Bloom County" comic strip. Copyright © 1985 by The Washington Post Writer's Group. Reprinted with permission.

Excerpt from *The Hero with a Thousand Faces* by Joseph Campbell, Bollingen Series XVII. Copyright 1949, © renewed 1976 by Princeton University Press. Reprinted by permission.

Photographs of asans and techniques by Charles Hudson, North Light Studio, Cleveland, Ohio.

Cartoon drawings on pp. 38, 158, 163, 168 and 184 by Kathy Detzer, Placerville, California.

Selected models' clothing furnished by:
Body 'n Soul, Cleveland, Ohio
Stripe Three, Inc., Cleveland, Ohio
Koenig Sporting Goods, Cleveland, Ohio.

The models for this book are all yoga students of the American Yoga Association.

THIS BOOK IS DEDICATED
TO RAMA,
THE SOURCE
FOR MY EXPRESSION
OF YOGA IN THE WORLD

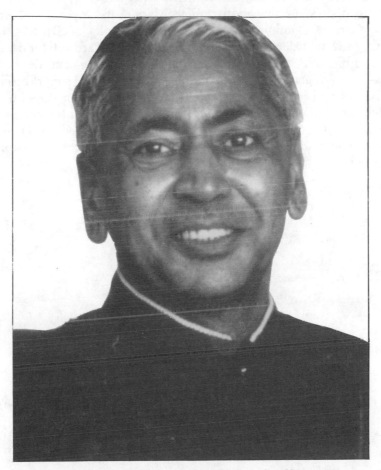

Swami Rama of Haridwar and Kashmir, India. 1900–1972

ACKNOWLEDGMENTS

The author wishes to thank the following people for their help in making this book a reality: Patricia Hammond for her substantial assistance in the writing and editing of the book; Jody Weiss and Cynthia Ingalls for their help in initiating the project; Thomas Ball for providing valuable advice about design; instructors Catherine Ball, Steve Gillum, Stephen Grant, Jane Holland, Cynthia Ingalls, James Kaplan, Nancy Leland, Deanna Muller, Mary Robison and Ed Wardwell for their extensive review of curriculum and techniques; the students who cheerfully and patiently served as models for the photographs: Mary Ann Doychak, Maureen Gillum, Corrine Goodman, Robin Lieberman, Polly McDowell, John Plassard, Michael Valentino and Frank Zatko; Anne Wardwell for detailed proofreading; and the many, many others—teachers, students and friends—who so generously gave of their time, effort and support to help produce this revision. Finally, special thanks go to Simon & Schuster's Eve Metz, head of design, and Bonni Leon, art director, for their creativity and hard work on this excellent production; and to editor Deborah Bergman, whose advice and encouragement have been a constant support throughout.

—ALICE CHRISTENSEN

CONTENTS

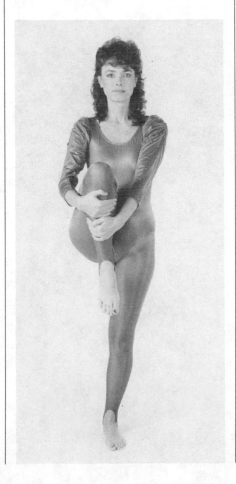

PREFACE

In the early fifties, when yoga first entered my life, hardly anyone knew anything at all about yoga, let alone practiced it. I did not even consciously seek yoga, as many people do today. Rather, yoga came to me with the suddenness of a vision one summer night and turned my life upside down.

I awoke out of a sound sleep to see a huge column of white light at the foot of my bed. Its radiance filled the room, reminding me of the intense light of downed power lines. I drew myself back against the headboard, terrified, but I could not speak or cry out. I knew that I was not dreaming, because I was aware of the curtains billowing softly at the open window and the maple tree waving gently outside in the summer breeze. I watched and waited, suddenly very quiet, as the light advanced toward me, covered me and seemed to enter me. I lost consciousness and awoke in the morning at my usual time. But as I got out of bed and started to dress, the word *yoga* sprang into my mind. I had only heard the word once before, at the annual county fair where one of the curiosities was a turbaned man who claimed to be able to foretell the future.

My life did not change much at first, except for the push of that word *yoga* in the back of my mind. I tried to approach the subject with other people, in roundabout ways, but I found no one who knew any more than I did. I found that it would not go away, so I started to read everything I could get my hands on in order to learn more about yoga. I even wrote to every yoga teacher and organization whose address I could find—but none of my letters was answered.

My life became more and more unsettling. I became clairvoyant. I started to dream in foreign languages and to have visions of strange people talking to me, teaching me things.

One man came more and more often in the visions and dreams— he was Swami Sivananda, then living at Rishikesh, in India. He began appearing to me at odd times, and at first I would run out of the room in fright. But eventually I lost my fear and my resistance to this upheaval in my life; I accepted this new work, and Sivananda began teaching me in earnest. Each day I spent several hours reading and studying, trying to meditate and trying to master the poses that I read about.

Yoga gave me tremendous concentration, and I found that I could continue to manage a large house and take care of my family even better than before. I became very efficient. Sorting out all the things in my life that I felt were not necessary, I settled down to concentrate on what had meaning for me and for those around me.

Sivananda taught me the beginnings of the techniques that have become the backbone of my life and thought. For several years he provided constant and sympathetic help in my search to find the meaning of yoga in my life. Just as I was making plans to go to India to meet him, I heard that Sivananda had died. Devastated, I tried to give up my yoga practices, only to find myself irresistibly drawn back to yoga and to its promises of health, peace, stability and true happiness in my life. I had found a wonderful acceptance in myself of who I was and what I could become, and the steadiness and support of that knowledge gave me the strength to continue what I knew I must do.

I kept on practicing, on my own, until I met Swami Rama of Kashmir and Haridwar, India, the next year. He was brought to this country by

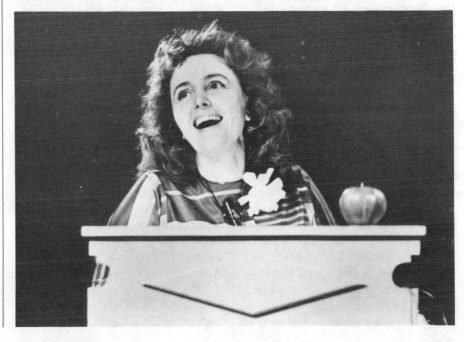

a group of people in Cleveland, where I lived. A student of his somehow found out about me (I never learned exactly how) and asked me to meet Rama at the airport. I will always remember his beautiful, clear brown laughing eyes looking into mine as he stepped off the plane in Cleveland and said, "Alice, I have come for you!" Rama became my guru—the teacher and guide whose love, inspiration and wisdom led me through the advanced training I needed to realize fully the possibilities that lay within me. Yoga had become a certainty in my life.

With Rama's guidance, the Light of Yoga Society (now known as the American Yoga Association) was formed in 1968 as a vehicle to make the benefits of yoga more easily accessible to people in this part of the world. Next, Rama oversaw the publication of the first edition of this book. And now, more than ten years after his death in 1972, I see many of his dreams taking shape as more and more people come to realize the freedom that yoga practice can bring about.

I have always wanted freedom: the freedom to find and to be myself; to do what I want to do in life and what I feel I *must* do. Yoga has given me that freedom. I no longer feel imprisoned by my fears, by ill health or by turbulent emotional swings. I no longer feel unable to communicate or to love. Yoga has enabled me to reach and explore new levels of awareness, so that my entire outlook on life has changed. I am happier now than I have ever been.

Several years ago I had the great good fortune to meet an old friend of Rama's in Kashmir: Swami Lakshmanjoo. This wonderful man, revered in India as a saint, is the only living master of a complex branch of yoga called Kashmir Shaivism. Lakshmanjoo has given

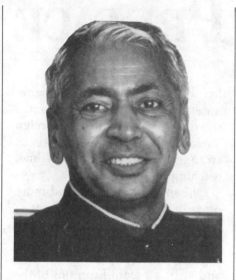

me the precious opportunity to continue being a student of yoga. In yoga the ability to keep learning is a rewarding quality. Life as a yogi is never boring! In all the years that have passed since that brilliant light first entered my life, I have been showered with the richness of new insight and experience. The results of my yoga practice and my teaching have not always been what I have expected, but they have always been what I most needed. Yoga has helped me attain that peace of mind, strength, inspiration and energy that all of us need for living a full and useful life.

In 1972, when the first edition of this book was published, our aim was to offer a clear and practical guide for people who were interested in finding out about yoga. The seventies were a time for trying out the many new attitudes and life-styles that seemed to offer a healthier and more fulfilling way of life than what America was used to. Yoga is one method of creating a sense of well-being that started out as fad but, in the eighties, has become recognized and appreciated as a dependable self-help source. Although very few people may feel drawn to practice yoga as intensively as I do, many more are beginning to recognize how even a

few yoga techniques, practiced regularly, can help us address the challenges and problems we face today.

Our world has become increasingly complex, filled with dismaying problems—such as famine, poverty and injustice— whose magnitude can inspire real feelings of helplessness. While we may often feel overwhelmed in the face of such global concerns, we *can* make a difference, starting with ourselves. By improving our health; by becoming more creative and productive, more aware of our motives and the effects of our actions, thoughts and desires; and by becoming less anxious or depressed, we become whole, happier with ourselves and with the challenges of daily life. That example cannot help but affect our community as well—family and friends, co-workers and even the strangers with whom we come into contact day after day. Happiness and well-being are contagious!

In the pages of this book you will find suggestions for using yoga to help make your life happier and more fulfilling. I wish you the best of success as you begin your adventure of yoga.

CHAPTER 1
HOW TO GET THE MOST OUT OF YOGA

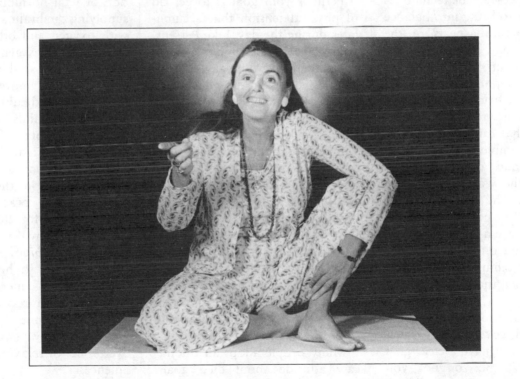

QUESTIONS COMMONLY ASKED ABOUT YOGA

Yoga is a step-by-step process that brings health, self-awareness and self-fulfillment. That process employs techniques that involve the body, the breath and the mind.

What Is the Purpose of Yoga?

The word *yoga* comes from the Sanskrit root "yug," which means "to join together" or "yoke." Yoga is a means to end the separateness that can exist internally between different aspects of yourself and externally, between yourself and the world. The techniques of yoga seek to bring into balance all the disparate aspects of the body, mind and personality, so that you end up with a strength and clarity of purpose supported by your whole being.

People come to yoga classes with goals that range from beginning a few simple stress management techniques to the desire to investigate the workings of their own minds. The adaptability of yoga makes it possible for students to achieve a variety of goals while pointing out new opportunities for stretching your horizons a little further than you thought you could.

As you start upon your adventure of self-discovery in yoga, you may or may not have a clear goal in mind. Whether or not you reach the goal you originally set out for, you will have learned a great deal about yourself along the way. And as your journey continues, your increased understanding and competence will make it easier to decide what you really want and to go for it!

Just for a moment, think of yourself as the hero in a mythological adventure. For example, imagine yourself as Perseus, the Greek hero who saved his love, Andromeda, and her city from a fearsome sea monster by turning the monster to stone with the head of Medusa. In order to find and bring back Medusa's head, Perseus had to recognize and win good advice from various helpers along the way, including Pegasus, the winged horse. He also had to overcome all sorts of obstacles and trials, facing great danger that tested his courage to the limit. He lost all his companions, endured harsh travel conditions and had to keep his wits about him in case of unexpected events. He really earned the title of champion!

Perhaps *your* goal is to get rid of physical tension that accumulates during the day. Like Perseus, your first task is to find out where to go for help. Your advisers (including your yoga teacher and/or this book) will help you discover where the tension is located in your body and which techniques will help you release it. Your daily techniques become your "armor" and the "weapons" you learn to use to attack and get rid of the physical tension. The obstacles you meet along the way could be a busy schedule that hampers your daily practice time, illness or procrastination, unexpected events, anxiety or depression that keep you from practicing; and so on.

Many people adopt an I-don't-care attitude about their goals, hoping to avoid disappointment if they don't get what they set out for. Because of their lack of commitment, they rarely achieve anything at all. The practice of yoga develops your capacity to achieve your goals, whatever they are; all you need is the willingness to practice regularly and observantly. Even ten minutes a day gives tremendous results!

What Techniques Does Yoga Use?

Yoga techniques focus on understanding and controlling the body, the breath and the mind through exercises (*asans*), breathing techniques (*pranayamas*) and meditation training.

Yoga *asans* (exercises) are designed to give maximum flexibility and strength to the skeletal, muscular and nervous systems, with special emphasis on building a strong and supple spine (to the capacity of each individual). Asans also massage internal organs and improve circulation, causing the release and distribution of vital hormones as well as supplying the brain and other cells with oxygen and other nutrients. Stretching asans gently work out muscle tension so that muscles are able to relax more easily. The gradual strengthening of the nervous system builds concentration, poise and a more stable emotional nature. (If you are interested in reading summaries of scientific studies relating to the physical effects of yoga practice, see the sources listed for this chapter in the Bibliography.)

Yoga *breathing* exercises are most effective in helping people cope with stress, increase their energy level and recover from fatigue. Also, controlled breathing will invariably have the spillover effect of relaxing mental turbulence.

Meditation practice helps you to consciously quiet the mental activity and emotional issues that constantly crowd the mind and enhances your ability to relax at will. Also, like many yoga students, you may find that meditation helps to periodically "clear the decks" in your mind and release dormant powers of intuition, creative methods of problem solving and other insights that can contribute to a clearer picture of yourself and the direction of your life.

Finally, you will find discussions of nutrition; stress management; the special concerns of athletes and pregnancy; and yoga philosophy that show how to make yoga practice part of an all-around healthier life-style.

Is Yoga a Religion?

Yoga is often mistakenly equated with Hinduism. Yoga actually predates Hinduism historically. It is a separate tradition of physical and psychological processes that lead to self-discovery.

Most people believe that there is a spiritual aspect to the personality along with the physical, mental, emotional and intuitive aspects. During the self-discovery process some people may decide to become better acquainted with this part of themselves and as a result become stimulated to renew or re-create their personal religious beliefs. Yoga does not prescribe a particular set of religious beliefs or, indeed, any at all. Rather, in students who pursue their acquaintance with their spiritual selves, the practice of yoga tends to enhance whatever traditions a person already possesses, adopts or renews.

Yoga tends to build a strong sense of self, through physical and emotional health and awareness; religion can supplement that awareness with a feeling of being more connected to the world, thus providing a reason for being. Also, as students find their awareness of themselves and the world around them increasing, they may experience feelings of appreciation and gratitude that religious traditions can help to express. In addition, the mental concentration and steadiness provided by yoga training help give a new meaning to old rituals, by improving the mind's ability to connect the symbol with the abstract idea that underlies it.

HOW TO GET THE MOST OUT OF YOGA PRACTICE

Use Your Common Sense

You should always check with your doctor before starting any new exercise program, especially if you have not exercised in several years. If you have physical limitations such as high blood pressure, heart disease, arthritis, spinal disk injuries or the like, take this book to your physician and ask his or her advice about which exercises you should avoid. If you have had surgery within the last two months, do not do any exercises until you have checked with your doctor.

Most people notice some minor soreness when they are beginning a new exercise program, especially after being inactive for a long time. However, severe pain in your back, legs or joints may indicate that you are pulling or straining too much in the exercises, or that you may have a severe physical problem that should be checked out with your physician immediately. If you notice severe pain, headaches, uncommon irritability, bleeding, muscle cramps, dislocations, dizziness or fainting, or other unusual symptoms, stop practicing until you are able to see your physician.

Even if you have practiced yoga before, we suggest that you start with the introductory routine for several weeks before launching into more difficult routines. Many times people experience an initial elation when they begin to practice yoga on a regular basis. This is due in part to the chemical changes, such as release of endorphins in the brain, that occur during any sustained exercise program, and in part to the special combination of movement, breathing and concentration that is unique to yoga. Be careful not to let your enthusiasm drive you to push or strain beyond your capacity. If you experience muscular pain and stiffness the day after exercising, that should indicate to you that you are doing too much. Set reasonable goals—both for the rate at which you progress through the lessons and for the amount of time each day you want to practice.

Warm up for at least five minutes before you go on to your first yoga asan routine. Remember to read through each exercise in Chapter 2 before trying it. If you have a physical limitation, you may need to modify the exercise in order to perform it comfortably. Remember to move slowly and deliberately, and not to strain. The benefit from doing asans lies not only in achieving a more limber body but in coordinating the physical movement with the breath pattern and a concentrated mind.

Chapter 3 on routines introduces suggested weekly course progressions. Go at your own pace. The weekly routines are suggestions only. If you are elderly or have physical limitations, proceed even more slowly than usual to give your body time to get used to the movements. You may have to simplify the positions somewhat. Be creative. Yoga is not a rigid process but a fluid one, allowing every individual to find his or her proper pace and intensity.

Competition is a word foreign to successful yoga practice. Try to think of your progress only in terms of yourself—not as compared to anyone else or even to the course sessions outlined in this book. You are an individual. If you go at your own pace, you will be practicing at just the right rate.

Similarly, don't be in a hurry to "convert" family and friends to yoga just because you are deriving so much benefit from it. The best way to show how something works is to demonstrate the results. When people around you start noticing that you are healthier, more in control, more rested and relaxed, and happier, the message will come across by itself!

Practice Regularly— But Enjoy It!

As in any new endeavor, practice makes perfect. The effects of yoga are cumulative. You will achieve the greatest—and longest-lasting —success in your practices if you make a commitment—a promise to yourself—to do some yoga techniques every day. Set reasonable goals. Establish the length of time that is comfortable and easy for you to stick with. Then any extra time you can add on a day-to-day basis will be icing on the cake. It is a good idea also to put together a minimum routine of three or four techniques for those exceptionally busy days that come up every so often.

If, like so many people, you are somewhat of a perfectionist, you may have the idea that if you don't have time to practice a full routine, you might as well not practice anything at all. Not true! In yoga the daily remembrance of practicing even a few minutes of the techniques will do wonders for building your concentration skills, improving your willpower and making it easier to do a little more the next day.

The time of day you choose to practice is totally up to you. Many people find that practicing first thing in the morning gives them a "wake-up" and a boost to start the day. Others cannot spare morning time and instead do their practices in the late afternoon or evening. An important point to remember is that you can split up the routine, for example, doing the exercises in the morning and the breathing and meditation in the evening. Whatever schedule you follow, try to stick with it long enough to see how it works —even on weekends.

It may take several weeks to discover your own optimal length of routine and times of day for yoga practice. But once you have, you will find it easier to stick to your practices. In fact, they will gradually become as habitual as brushing your teeth. This steadiness of practice will pay off by carrying you through those times when it seems like you aren't making much progress at all— what we call the deserts. At first the effects of yoga practice are many and obvious, and you will experience elation at being more well and relaxed than you've ever been. After several weeks or months of practice, however, the effects start to become more subtle and less noticeable on the surface. If you can keep going steadily during those times, you will be rewarded by even better, and longer-lasting, results.

SETTING YOURSELF UP

Clothing

Wear clothing that is loose and/or stretchy, such as an exercise suit with elastic or drawstring waist, or a leotard. (See Chapter 10 for techniques you can do at the of-fice, in line at the store, and so on, which require no change of clothes.) Dress for the season and the temperature of your house, but be sure you are warm enough. Wear socks but not shoes. When you get ready to do the meditation, have a sweater, a blanket or something to throw over yourself because your body temperature will tend to drop as you relax. Also, it is important to practice yoga in a draft-free room.

Equipment

Have a blanket, mat or large towel at hand *even if your room is carpeted.* Reserve this blanket exclusively for your yoga practices —along with your exercise clothes—as this will help reinforce the consistency of regular daily practice.

For seated breathing you will need one or more throw cushions or pillows. You may want to experiment with several different kinds or combinations of pillows to find the right degree of height and comfort. (See further discussion of posture on pp. 132-33).

Environment

Try to avoid interruptions while you practice yoga. If you are able, turn your phone off (at *least* during meditation) or put a sign on your bedroom door so that you won't be disturbed. You deserve this time for yourself. With communication and patience you will be able to work out a schedule that harmonizes with your work and family responsibilities. When you are on vacation or in a different environment, work out an alternative place and time so that you get a little time to yourself. Learn to enjoy your privacy.

At the office think about taking a few minutes during the day to practice a few techniques you have learned. You'll probably find the breathing especially helpful. (See Chapter 10, Yoga and Stress Management, for more suggestions.) If you don't have access to a private office or a private space, consider the broom closet, rest room or supply room for a three-minute getaway!

Cautions About Drugs

Never do yoga while under the influence of alcohol or recreational drugs. Recreational drugs should be completely avoided—it is very dangerous to mix yoga with drug use.

By disrupting biochemically the normal neurological pathways to the brain, drugs do indeed change a person's consciousness, but in the process they also destroy concentration. Nothing could be more devastating to the practice of classical yoga, which has never been rivaled in the field of mental concentration and its subtleties. The ability to focus the mind voluntarily on an object without interruption for extended periods of time (called *ekagrata*) is the single most valuable tool of yoga. Indeed, concentration is the very basis for all learning and education and should be protected and developed, not destroyed by drugs. As if that were not enough, paranoia and loss of personal motivation are further tragic results of drug use.

Depending on drugs to "do it for you" makes you lose your ability to control and shape your own mental/emotional life; as a result, you become psychologically dependent on external methods of affecting the way you feel inside. In yoga you learn to do something for yourself through your own steady practice of mental and physical techniques. The inner focus and control these

practices develop make you healthier, more flexible and adaptive and, therefore, better able to cope with the stresses of life.

If you are in the habit of using drugs—even infrequently—we suggest that you try an experiment for a few weeks and quit completely while you start yoga practice. You will probably find that you no longer feel the need or desire for the drugs, because you will gain better and longer-lasting benefits.

If you are taking prescription medications, by all means follow your doctor's instructions. However, certain medications, such as large doses of tranquilizers, can affect your success with yoga. If you are in doubt, ask your physician.

A Word About Addictions

Many authorities view addiction (the psychological and/or physical craving for something) as a misguided response to stress. In other words, the body and mind are trying to get a message across about some need, but it is interpreted and translated into a need for an easier substitute.

If you find yourself addicted to cigarettes, alcohol, sugar, caffeine or other substances, you may find that practicing yoga can help by giving you alternative ways of responding to stress. Yoga will help improve your willpower, strengthen your nervous system, teach you how to relax at will and give you tools for more constructively handling the stresses in your life. Heavy smokers may experience dizziness during some exercise or breathing, due to reduced lung capacity. If that is the case for you, reduce multiple repetitions of the techniques. See the chapter on nutrition for nutrients that can help fight addictions.

Yoga and Other Forms of Exercise

Many people ask if it is beneficial to combine yoga with other physical activities such as jogging, dancing or weight training. It is certainly a good idea to be as physically active as you like to be. It is also good to balance the passive stretches of yoga asans and relaxation training with aerobic conditioning, since yoga asans do not (at least at the introductory level) provide that. Later in this book you will find several routines that can be used to provide essential warm-up and cool-down stretches to limber muscles and tendons and prevent injuries.

Food and Drink

It is a good idea to wait for from one to one and a half hours after eating before practicing yoga asans. However, if you are really hungry at the time you wish to exercise, or if it has been several hours since you last ate, have a light snack (yogurt, fruit, cottage cheese, a small salad, soup or a piece of bread) to tide you over. (See Chapter 7, Yoga and Nutrition, for other suggestions for nutritious snacks.)

The main reason for not exercising immediately after eating is that a full stomach will feel very uncomfortable as you bend and compress. It will also be harder to breathe deeply. The process of digestion temporarily diverts blood flow from other areas of the body to your stomach, which is why you may feel sluggish, sleepy or unable to concentrate well after eating. For this reason you may also find that it is harder to quiet your mind in meditation when you are full.

Because of its stimulation of the central nervous system, caffeine acts somewhat like a trigger for a stress response in your body. We therefore recommend that you try to follow the same time interval for caffeine as for food.

FINDING A YOGA TEACHER

In some ways finding a yoga teacher in the United States today is much easier than when yoga was first developing—now all you have to do is go to the phone book or bookstore and you have hundreds of potential teachers from whom to choose. The real problem is how to find a *good* yoga teacher, especially when you don't know much about yoga yourself.

As yet, unfortunately, there is no nationally recognized standard for certification of yoga teachers; some organizations may grant certification after attendance at a week-long workshop, and others may require several years. When you write or call to find a teacher in your area, don't be afraid to ask about qualifications; a good teacher will not mind your questions. Following are a few suggestions based on our standards at the American Yoga Association.

Find out whether the teacher practices yoga exercise, breathing and meditation as a *daily* discipline or just occasionally as one of a number of other activities. Find out if the teacher *studies regularly with a teacher* of his or her own. This is important, because no matter how long someone has been practicing yoga, he or she never outgrows the need to keep learning. Yoga is a continual learning process. No one becomes so proficient in a given number of months or years that he or she doesn't need a teacher anymore. American Yoga Association

teachers are all committed to daily practice and attend a regular class as students in addition to a regular teacher training class.

A genuine teacher has allowed yoga concepts to *influence his or her life-style.* Teachers should be vegetarian. They should not smoke at all, or use recreational drugs. They should be nutritionally aware, following guidelines such as those outlined in this book. Their conduct should be responsible, safe and aware, based on the ethical guidelines set forth by Patanjali (see Chapter 11, Philosophies for Life).

A good yoga teacher has spent time *studying the various effects of yoga exercises, breathing, and meditation*; has a *working knowledge of major muscle groups and body systems*; and is *able to vary the techniques according to each person's individual capability.* A genuine yoga teacher also will not confuse the yoga techniques by allowing his or her own religious beliefs to affect the class.

These guidelines may be strict, but at the American Yoga Association we believe that teachers of yoga must be exceptionally conscientious and professional in their work of transmitting to others the exacting disciplines of yoga. These personal commitments ensure that teachers avoid any injury or misrepresentation in their classes.

If you are interested in having American Yoga Association teachers come to your area for a program, please write to us at this address:
American Yoga Association
P.O. Box 18487
Cleveland, OH 44118–0487

HOW TO PRACTICE YOGA ASANS

Read the Introduction

Before anything else, *read this complete introduction* and all cautions. Check with your doctor before starting any new exercise program.

Always Warm Up

Always warm up before starting a routine. If you have a limited time schedule, do the first half of the warm-up routine only (through the Lazy Stretch exercise).

Follow Curriculum and Instructions

At the American Yoga Association we feel that yoga is best approached in a holistic manner, with a complete program of exercise, breathing and meditation. Following this introduction you will read a section on warming up, with a complete routine that should be followed by everyone, regardless of your level of proficiency. After that we will outline a curriculum of three courses, each ten weeks in length, approximating the format of our actual classes. For best results from your yoga practice, follow the curriculum as outlined and include some exercise, breathing and meditation in each practice session. You can always cut down on your total practice time if you have a tight schedule. To help you remember which exercises go with which course, each exercise in the Exercise (Asans) chapter is marked with a Roman numeral *I* for Course One, *II* for Course Two and *III* for Course Three.

When you have warmed up and are ready to start the actual asans, read the instructions through once. Then try the exercise, following· the illustrations. Reread the instructions to make sure you have followed them correctly. Especially note the breath instructions with each exercise. If you practice yoga without paying attention to correct breathing, you will become quite limber but you will miss some of the subtler effects of yoga asans that are brought about by the various breath patterns. (A more complete description of the breath patterns evident in all yoga asans can be found in the description of Course Two in Chapter 3.) Then repeat the exercise the given number of times.

Breathe Deeply and Slowly

In most exercises you will be instructed to breathe deeply and slowly. Do not hold your breath except where specified, and at no time should you hold your breath in or out for more than five seconds.

Always breathe in and out through your nose while exercising, unless your physician has specifically advised you to breathe out through your mouth. Breathing through the nose (besides filtering out many impurities and germs in the air) helps you maintain important control over the length and smoothness of your breath.

Move Slowly and Deliberately

Be sure you are moving slowly, carefully and smoothly in the asans. Remember that the *process* of moving through an exercise is just as important as the *goal* of attaining a particular position. In fact, we believe that limberness, as a goal in itself, is less important than the goal of becoming more aware of how your body works and what it needs in order to become healthier and stronger.

Never bounce, jerk or bend quickly as you exercise. In yoga you are stretching and strengthening very delicate nerve and muscle tissue, so move gently, and be aware of areas of special strain or tension so you don't hurt yourself. Another important reason not to bounce is that as you progress in yoga, you will be instructed to hold various positions at times, breathing gently. This hold greatly increases the effectiveness of the exercise.

Repetitions

Except for the warm-up sequence, yoga asans are to be repeated no more than three times. This is because of their tremendous effectiveness. We recommend that you do your routine only once each day. Practicing an asan routine more than once a day may overstimulate your nervous system, making you tense, irritable or high-strung. If you want to exercise at another time of day, do some aerobic conditioning instead.

Rest Periodically

After every three or four asans, rest for a minute or so in either the Standing Rest Pose, the Corpse Pose, the Baby Pose or the East Bridge Rest (all described on pp. 52-53) Completely relax so you go limp. Try not to think too much about what you are going to do next; just let your body rest.

Balance and Limberness Vary

Because your body is so greatly affected by how well you cope with stress, how much sleep you are getting, how balanced and regular your diet is and many other factors, you will find that your limberness and sense of balance will vary slightly from day to day. Also, everyone is much stiffer in the morning than in the afternoon or evening. Do not be discouraged by these slight variations; if you practice daily you will notice a steady overall progression despite occasional variations. The important thing to remember is to be regular in your practices.

Don't Exercise When Ill

Do not exercise when you are ill, even if you have "just a cold." No matter how "common" the illness, your body needs rest most of all—not more demands. In some instances, such as with a sinus infection or head cold, exercising may even spread the infection or at least worsen your symptoms.

Special Notes for Women Only

We strongly advise you not to practice strenuous yoga asans during your menstrual period. The main reason for this is that most yoga asans impose some pressure or stretch on the abdominal area, and this can increase bleeding. Also, the stimulation yoga exercises give to your hormonal system, combined with the natural hormonal changes happening during your period, may cause you to experience increased nervousness, irritability or upset. Course I includes an alternate routine for you to practice during that time so that you can be active but still safe (see p. 37). We also encourage you to add exercises from other types of activities, such as aerobic dance or calisthenics, using these guidelines:

1. Do not perform exercises that compress the abdomen either by extreme forward or extreme backward bending.
2. Do not perform inverted (upside-down) exercises.
3. Do not hold the breath.
4. Do not perform exercises that

require abdominal strength, such as sit-ups.

NURSING MOTHERS

For similar reasons we suggest that nursing mothers refrain from yoga practice until their babies have been completely weaned. We feel that the hormonal changes brought about by yoga practice are evident in the chemical composition of the mother's milk and are not suitable for the well-being of the child.

PREGNANCY

If you are pregnant you may do a limited routine of asans *after the first trimester* if there have been no complications and your physician approves. See Chapter 8, Yoga During Pregnancy, for special routines for you. You may find that yoga in the last six months of your term may help you have an easier delivery and a more relaxed, happier baby. If you decide to take Lamaze classes, you will find that yoga harmonizes with those techniques very well.

CHAPTER 2

GETTING READY TO EXERCISE: THE YOGA WARM-UP

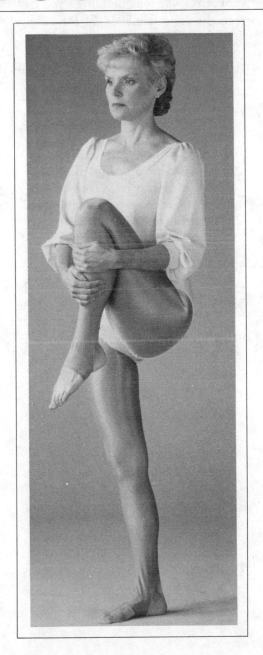

WARMING UP

Now you are ready to begin practicing yoga by first learning to warm up properly. Before you start make sure you have read the introduction of this book in Chapter 1 thoroughly and understand all the cautions and suggestions. A complete curriculum for three ten-week courses is outlined in the next chapter. It would be a good idea to read over Chapter 3, Curriculum and Routines, in order to get an idea of how the techniques all fit together.

In the weekly curriculum lists the warm-up exercises are not listed separately but as a group: the "warm-up sequence." After a few weeks of practice you will probably know the warm-ups so well that you will not have to refer back to the description of each exercise in this chapter.

Whether you are a total beginner or have practiced for several years, you still should warm up before every session, using the warm-up sequence that follows. It is vitally important to start every day's routine with a warm-up sequence. Warming up has nothing to do with the temperature of the room or how limber your body may feel already. In yoga exercise you'll be working not only with the large muscle groups, but also with delicate nerves, connective tissue, blood vessels and internal organs. Warming up allows you to ready your whole body for exercise, so that it begins easily and without a lot of fear or tension. If you are rushed or especially tense, you may want to spend extra time warming up or even use the sequence as your complete exercise commitment for the day.

Warming up is also an opportunity to warm up your mind—in other words, to relax your mind, quiet extraneous thoughts and center yourself where you are, instead of letting your mind wander. All yoga asans affect particular areas of the body. In your warm-up sequence begin the process of doing an exercise in such a way that you use only the muscle groups that are required by the asan—keep the rest relaxed. Warming up stimulates your kinesthetic sense—your sense of where your body is in space.

As you warm up, pay attention to what your body is saying to you. Is it expressing tension or pain anywhere? Is it fatigued, strained, ill or angry? Learn to listen for your body's signals; you'll learn more about how your body works, how it reacts, what it needs. Remember this concept when you begin to do more vigorous exercises; your body will resist growth with pain if it is forced or bullied; a gentle approach yields positive changes much more quickly because there is much less fear.

SHOULDER ROLLS

Limbers shoulder joints
Reduces tension in upper back and neck muscles
Improves posture
Relieves arthritic stiffness and pain in shoulder joints

Stand with arms at your sides. Let them hang loose just like wet spaghetti (A). Lift both shoulders up toward your ears (B), then roll them in a circle forward (C), down, back (D) and then up toward your ears again. Repetitions: 3 to 5 each direction. Breathe normally; don't hold your breath. To help loosen and relax especially stiff shoulders, massage your shoulder and neck before and after this exercise. After all repetitions, shake out your arms to relax them.

• Keep arms and hands limp.
• Breathe normally.

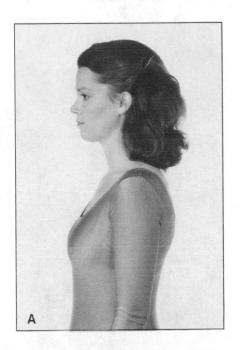

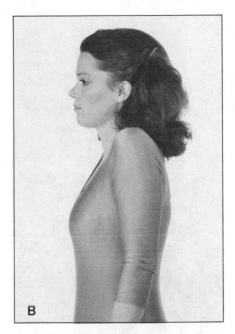

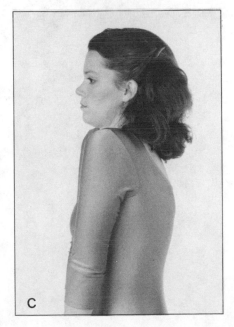

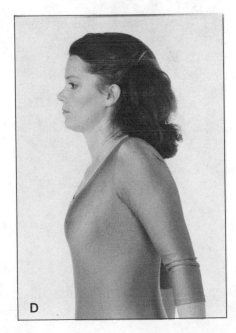

ELBOW TOUCH

Limbers shoulder joints
Reduces tension in upper and mid-back muscle groups
Improves posture

Bend your elbows so that your fingers touch your shoulders. Slowly bring your elbows together in front (A), then horizontally to the sides and to the back (B), squeezing your shoulder blades together. Breathe normally. Don't hold your breath. Repetitions: 3 to 5.

• Breathe normally.
• Keep elbows horizontal to floor.

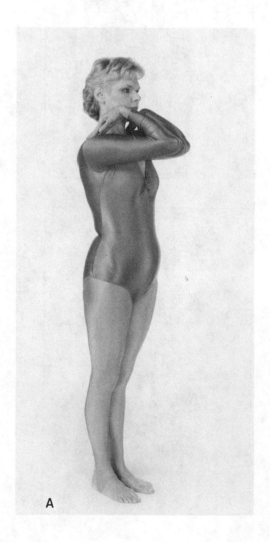

A

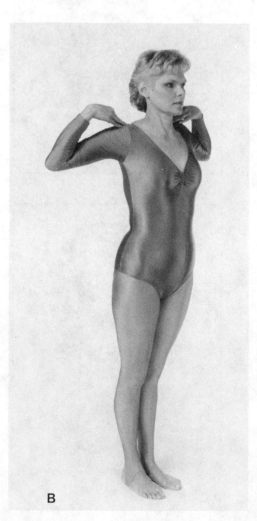

B

ARM ROLLS

Limbers shoulder joints
Stretches and strengthens upper back muscles
Stimulates nerves in the arms
Improves circulation in torso, neck and head

Raise your arms parallel to the floor. Flex your hands back toward your head, as if stopping traffic to your left and right (A). Now start rotating your arms forward in large circles, having hands almost touch in front (B), and rotating as far back as your shoulder joint will allow (C). Move slowly. Breathe normally. Repetitions: 3 to 5 circles forward, then 3 to 5 backward. Keep fingers flexed stiffly during the entire movement, and keep elbows straight.

Relax arms to sides and shake out shoulders, arms and lower back by wiggling like a limp rag doll all over, to relax the muscles and nerves.

Continue with smaller, faster circles out to the sides, making circles about the size of a dinner plate. Remember to do the same number of circles in both directions.

Note: If you have high blood pressure or heart disease (and assuming that you have your doctor's permission to practice yoga), do not attempt the smaller rotations until you have practiced the large ones for several months, since the smaller rotations put extra strain on the heart muscles. (You will probably notice that the extra circulation pumping brought about by this exercise will make your upper body feel warm and flushed.) Check with your doctor if you have any doubts about what you should or should not do.

- Keep fingers flexed and elbows straight.
- Breathe normally.
- Make large circles as big as possible; small ones the size of dinner plates.

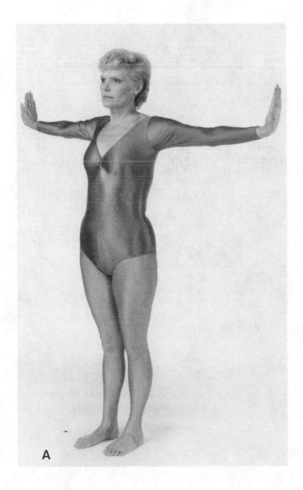

A

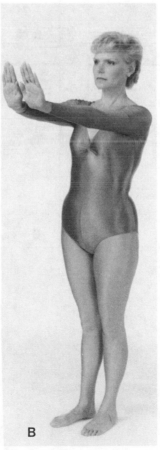

B

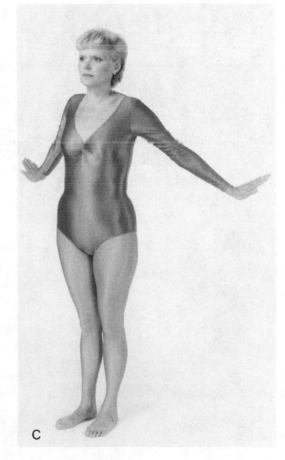

C

NECK STRETCH

Limbers the neck and improves circulation in the throat
Reduces tension in the neck muscles
Limbers the cervical spine

There are several options for arm positions in this exercise. We recommend that you start with your arms parallel to the floor, palms up. If this is too fatiguing, you can rest your hands on your hips or let them hang at your sides. Choose the position that best helps you keep your shoulders from tensing or lifting as you move your head around. In this exercise only the neck muscles are involved—and the rest of your body should remain relaxed.

Start by lowering your chin to your chest(A); then lift your chin up so you are looking up at the ceiling (B). (Avoid dropping head all the way back because of the extra strain this causes on the neck.) Repetitions: 3, breathing normally.

Next, starting with head straight, tilt head to the right side, ear over your shoulder (C), then lift your head up and gently tilt over toward the opposite (left) shoulder (D). Try not to lift your shoulder up toward your ear, but move only the head. Breathe normally. Repetitions: 3.

Next, starting again with head straight, turn and look over your

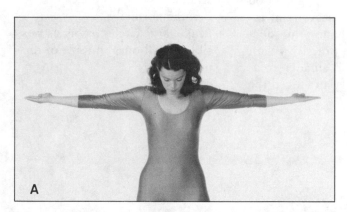

A

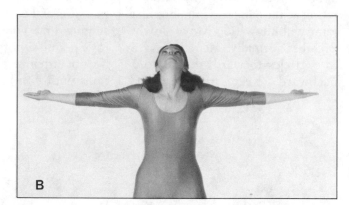

B

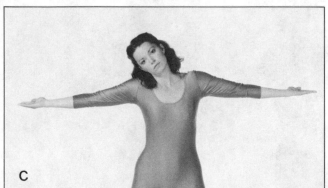

C

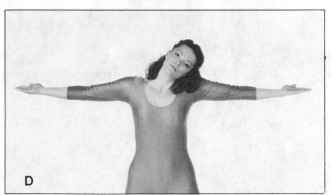

D

right shoulder (E), then your left (F). Repetitions: 3.

Note: If you have any kind of neck problem or injury, including occasional neck pain, *stop here*. If not, go on to the final two variations.

This next variation moves your neck in a gentle semicircle back and forth. Start by lowering your chin to your chest (A). Slowly roll your head to the right until you reach the right "tilt" position: ear over shoulder, face forward (C). Roll back down to your chest and over to your left (D), then continue the back-and-forth roll for a total of three complete repetitions.

If the variation gives your neck no problem, go on to the final variation: Starting with your chin lowered to your chest (A), slowly rotate your head to the right, ear above shoulder (C), remembering to keep shoulders relaxed throughout; then roll your head up and over to the left shoulder (D) and finally roll forward to your starting position. Relax your arms and shake them out. Repetitions: 3 in each direction.

- Keep lips and teeth together.
- Breathe normally.
- Don't lift shoulders.
- Move slowly.
- Don't drop head far back.

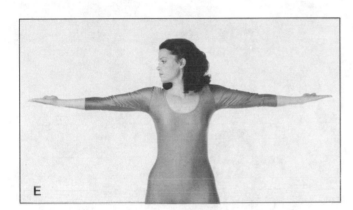

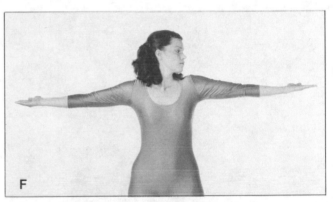

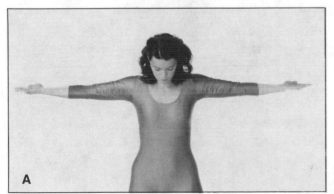

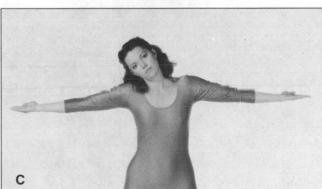

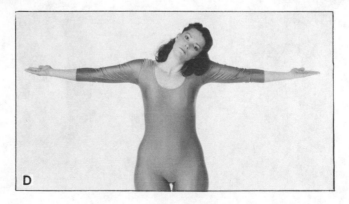

STANDING REACH

*Limbers and strengthens shoulder
    joints*
Expands rib cage
Strengthens ankles and calves
Improves balance

Standing with your arms at your sides, breathe out completely (A). Fix your gaze on a spot on the floor or wall—this will help you keep your balance. Now start to breathe in, at the same time bringing your arms up in a wide circle to the sides and overhead while coming up on your toes (B). Hold your breath for just a second as you clasp hands and stretch a little farther up toward the ceiling. Then breathe out while returning straight arms to the sides and down, and lower heels to floor. Repetitions: 3.

On days when your balance is less steady, divide the exercise in two: first, breathe in and lift arms out to the sides and up overhead, clasp hands and stretch, then breathe out and down. Next, holding on to a chair or bar for balance, breathe in and come up on toes, then breathe out and lower heels to floor. Repetitions: 3 for each part.

• Stare at one spot for balance.
• Breathe deeply through your nose.

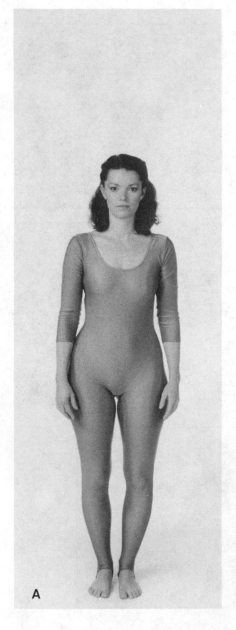

A

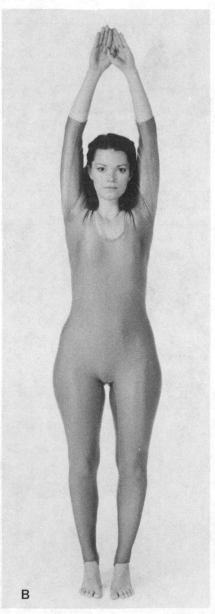

B

EASY BEND

Limbers upper back muscles and shoulder joints
Improves circulation to head
Relieves tension in upper back and neck
Gives a light stretch to the muscles and nerves in the legs, back and neck

Stand straight, with feet parallel, arms at sides (A). Breathe out. Now breathe in and raise your arms up at the same time, until they are outstretched, parallel to the floor (B). Your chest should be fully expanded. Now start to breathe out and slowly "dive" forward into a slouch, letting your head and arms relax completely (C). Bend only halfway (even if you can easily bend much farther) so that your hands hang down at about the level of your knees. Your breath should now be completely out. Now start to breathe in as you lift slowly back to a standing position, bringing your arms up and out to the sides again and rolling your spine up from the bottom. Then begin breathing out and bending forward as you continue repetitions in a kind of pumping motion, breathing out as you bend forward and breathing in as you straighten up. Try to match your breath to your movement so that your exhalation lasts for the whole movement forward and your inhalation lasts for the whole movement back up. Repetitions: 3. After the last inhalation, just breathe out and relax, slowly lowering arms to sides.

- Breathe through your nose.
- Try to match your breath to your movement.
- Relax head, neck, arms and hands completely in the forward position.
- Move slowly and deliberately—but not so slowly that you start gasping for breath.

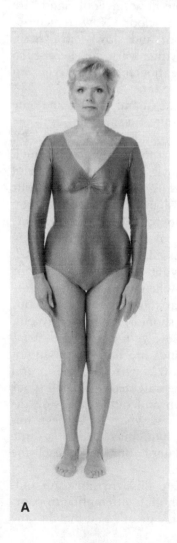

A

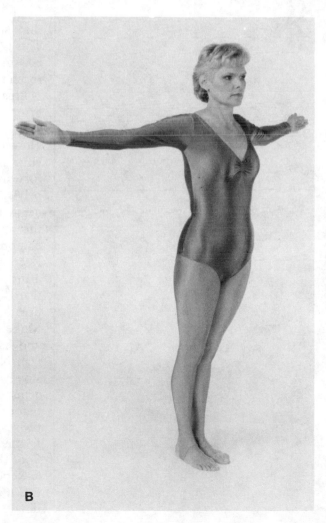

B

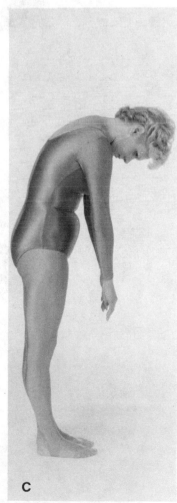

C

LAZY STRETCH

Stretches the back of the legs
Begins to limber the lower back
Stretches chest muscles

With your feet parallel and a few inches apart, bend your knees a little and place your elbows on your knees with hands clasped. Lift your head slightly and breathe in (A). Now breathe out, tuck your head and straighten your legs as much as possible, keeping elbows in place (B). Repetitions: 3 to 5.

- Coordinate breath and movement.
- Don't stretch to the point of discomfort.
- Remember to lift head on inhalation and tuck on exhalation.

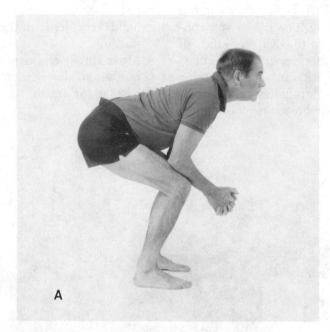

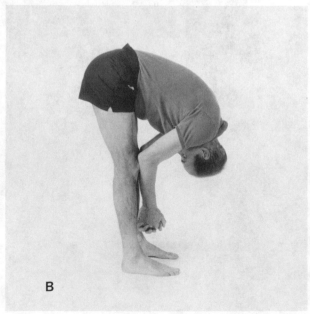

FULL BENDS

Stretches nerves and muscles along the back of the legs and spine all the way up to the back of the head, helping heal sciatic nerve problems and varicose veins
Improves circulation to entire body
Strengthens rib cage, lungs and heart
Strengthens postural muscles
Strengthens lower back

This exercise begins similarly to the Easy Bend. Start with feet parallel, arms at sides (A). Before you begin, first just bend forward gently without bending your knees and note how far your hands are from the floor. Now remember that spot and slowly straighten. This is still a warm-up exercise, so be sure not to strain trying to reach too far.

Breathe in and at the same time bring your arms up and out to the sides, expanding your chest (B). Now start to breathe out (through your nose, remember) and bend forward from the hips, tilting your pelvis slightly forward as you begin to bend (C). This prevents the spinal vertebrae from being compressed and possibly injured. Keep your head between your arms. When you have bent forward as far as you can, your breath should be all the way out. Make sure your neck, head, arms and hands are limp at this point (D). Now start to breathe in and slowly straighten, bringing your arms up and out to the sides as before. As your limberness improves, you may stretch a little farther until your hands reach the floor (E).

Repeat this rhythmic up-and-down motion, attempting to coordinate the breath so it matches the movement. It may take a few weeks to learn to do this, but it is essential for a smooth movement. Try to move slowly, but not so slowly that you start gasping for breath. A breath length of about five seconds should be comfortable for most people in the beginning. Try counting as you bend for a few days until you learn the correct speed. Repetitions: 3 to 5.

- Coordinate breath with movement.
- Move slowly and deliberately.
- Don't strain to reach the floor.
- Breathe through your nose.

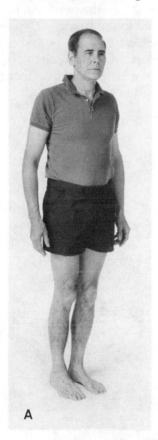

A

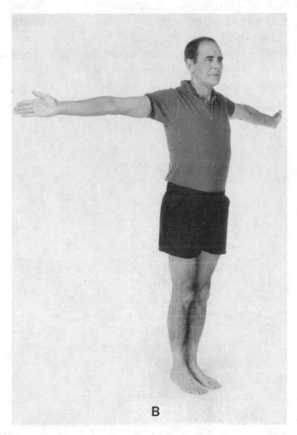

B

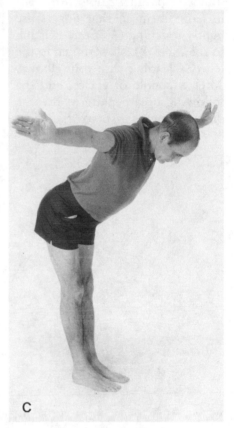

C

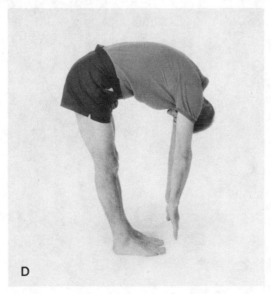

D

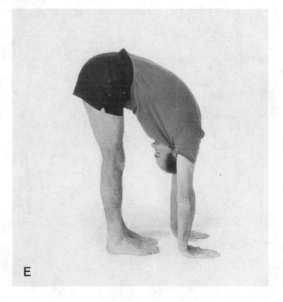

E

ELBOW TWIST

Improves flexibility in the spinal column

Relieves tension in the upper back and shoulders

With feet separated a few inches (but still parallel), hold arms out in front, bent so that fingers are lightly touching (A). Start twisting to the right (B), slowly, then to the left (C), leading with your elbows. After a couple of cycles, add the following breath pattern: Breathe *out* as you twist to the side, breathe *in* as you return to the front, breathe *out* to the other side, breathe *in* to the front, and so on. Keep your arms bent and back straight, concentrating on the gentle sideways twisting motion of your spine. Repetitions: 3 to 5 in each direction.

In this exercise your head should turn with your body so that there is no extra twist to the neck. For a variation, however, you can have your head turn the opposite way from your arms.

(Do not do this variation if you have disk problems in your neck.) Another variation is to raise your arms overhead and lower them to your waist as you twist.

- Breathe *out* into the twist and *in* going back to the front.
- Keep the rest of your body relaxed (especially stomach!).
- Try to twist from the hip rather than from the knees.

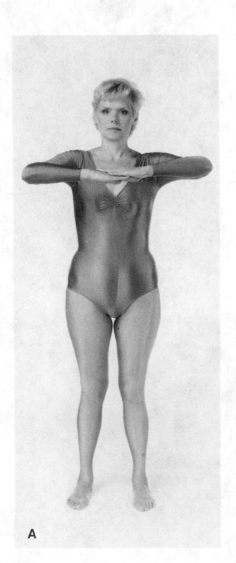

A

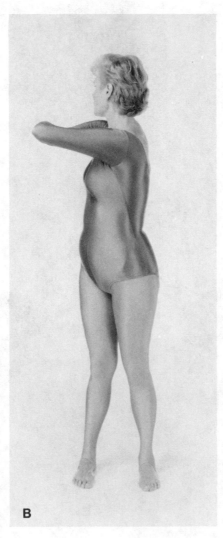

B

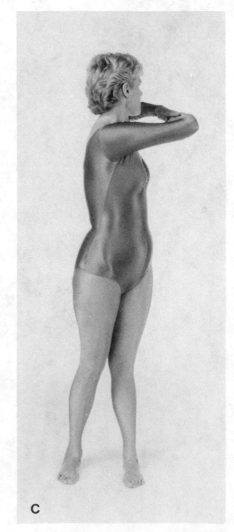

C

LEG LIFTS

Strengthens and tones leg muscles
Improves balance
Stretches back of legs
Improves circulation in legs, urinary tract and reproductive organs

Start with both hands on your hips. Extend your left arm straight out in front of you. Keeping *both knees straight*, lift the right leg up toward your hand, with toes flexed toward your face (A). The speed should be somewhere between a kick and a lift. Keep breath relaxed. Most important, keep legs straight! This is much more important than reaching your hand with your toes.

Note that you are lifting the *opposite* leg toward your hand. Repetitions: 3 to 5.

Switch sides so that your right arm is extended, and lift the left leg up. Repetitions: 3 to 5. Keep your other arm on your hip, for balance. On days when your balance is shaky, hold on to a chair back instead of having the hand on your hip.

Now extend your left arm out to the side and lift your left leg (B), noting that you are now lifting the leg on the *same side* as the extended arm. Instead of "turning out" your leg, as in ballet, so that your toes point to the ceiling, keep your foot pointed forward so that

you will lift and strengthen the muscles and nerves along the sides of your hips and legs. Repetitions: 3 to 5. Switch to right side and repeat.

Then, with both hands on your hips, lift each leg slowly backward, keeping knees straight (C). Don't lean forward, but instead use your back and buttock muscles to lift the leg. Try not to bend your knee as you lift. Repetitions: 3 to 5 each leg.

- Breathe normally.
- Keep knees straight and toes flexed at all times.
- Keep torso straight.

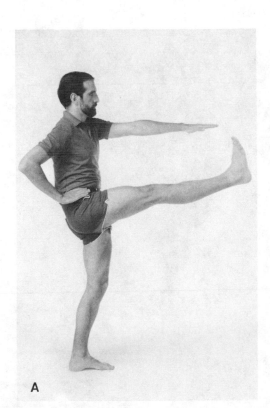

A

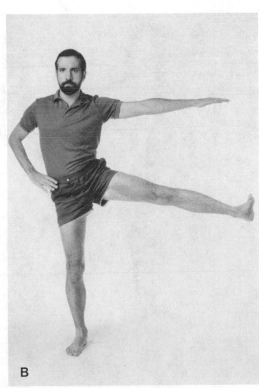

B

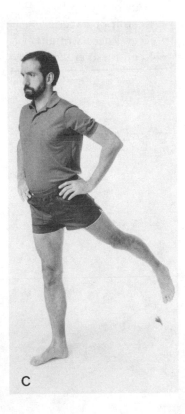

C

COMPLETE LEG LIFTS: Variation

Strengthens hip joints and lower back
Improves balance
Strengthens nerves and tones muscles in legs and hips
Removes fatty deposits from thighs, hips, buttocks and waist

Standing with both hands on hips, slowly raise one leg to the front, keeping toes flexed and knees straight. Stare at one spot and breathe normally. Now, keeping your foot raised, slowly move it out to the side, toes pointed forward, then to the back, trying not to lean forward to compensate. Return your foot to the floor. Using the same leg, reverse direction, starting by lifting your leg to the back, then to the side, then to the front. Repeat in both directions with opposite leg.

- Breathe normally. Don't hold your breath.
- Keep foot flexed.
- Keep knees straight.
- Keep torso erect.

STANDING KNEE SQUEEZE

Improves functioning of digestive system
Limbers hip joints and knees
Strengthens back and legs
Improves balance and circulation
Relieves lower back tension

Stand with feet parallel. Breathe out. Now breathe in as you raise your right knee. Hold your breath in as you squeeze the knee in toward your body with both hands (A). (Remember to stare at one spot for balance.) Let your foot relax rather than flex. Then relax, breathe out, and lower your leg to the floor.

After a few days, add the following variation: After releasing your compression, grasp your leg at the ankle and squeeze the leg to the back while exhaling (B). (Note: If you have arthritis in your knees or an injury that is painful if you squeeze your knee, then grasp your thigh instead, just underneath your knee. You'll get the same effect of the compression on your stomach without the strain on your knee joint.) Repetitions: 3 each leg, alternating.

On days when your balance is less steady, hold on to a chair back with one hand and squeeze the lifted knee with the other (C), or lean your back or side against a wall.

- Stare at one spot.
- Hold complete breath in while squeezing the knee.
- Relax foot.

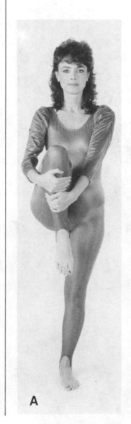

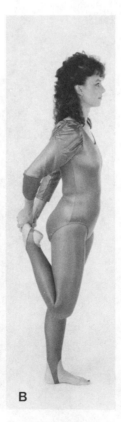

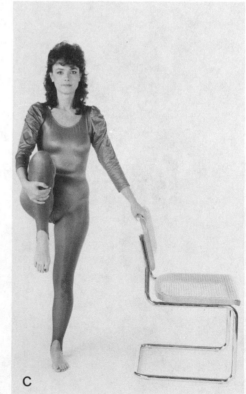

A　　B　　C

MASSAGE KNEES AND ANKLES

Warms and relaxes knee and ankle joints

Sit on the floor with legs in front. Massage each knee (A) and ankle (B) for several seconds with both hands. Rub lightly, using your whole hands, until the joint feels warm. (Note: Rubbing your joints regularly with oil or lotion will help them limber up more quickly.)

Rotate ankles several times in circles each way.

• Use your whole hand when massaging—not just your fingers.

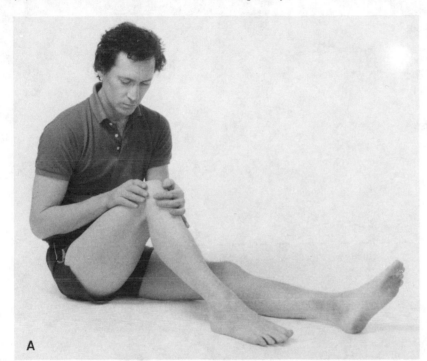

A

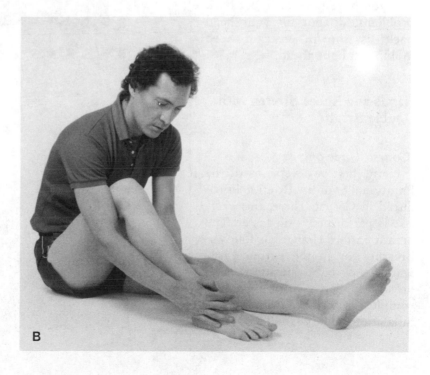

B

HANDS AND KNEES STRETCH

Limbers lower back
Stretches chest muscles
Loosens hip and knee joints

Sitting on your feet on the floor, breathe out. Then start to breathe in and come forward so that you are on all fours (A). Then simply lower your hips a little and look up, keeping your arms stiff (B). Breathe out and sit back on your feet, bending forward with arms still out in front (C). Breathe in and move forward again. Repetitions: 3 to 5.

- Keep arms straight.
- Look up on inhalation.

Note: If you have trouble sitting on your feet due to knee or ankle problems, start the exercise on hands and knees and just rock slightly back on the exhalation as far as you can without strain, instead of sitting all the way back on your feet.

If you have neck or upper back problems, do not tilt your head back as shown; instead, keep looking straight ahead.

Hands and Knees Stretch with Double Breath

(Course Three only)
In the first two versions of the Emotional Stability Routine introduced in Course Three, this exercise is performed a bit faster. The breath pattern changes as follows: Breathe *out* in the extreme forward and back positions and breathe *in* between, so that each complete repetition includes two inhalations and two exhalations.

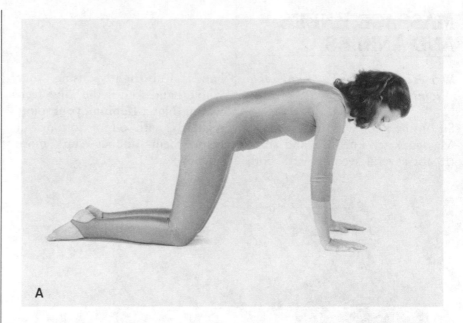

A

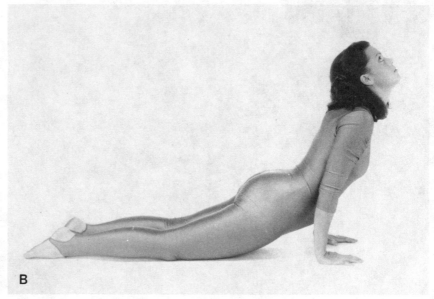

B

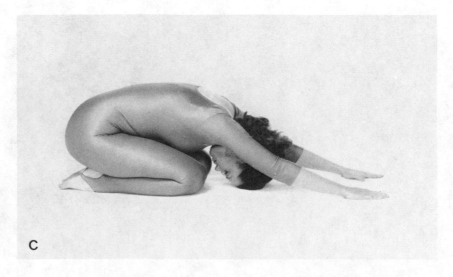

C

CHAPTER 3
PUTTING IT ALL TOGETHER: CURRICULUM AND ROUTINES

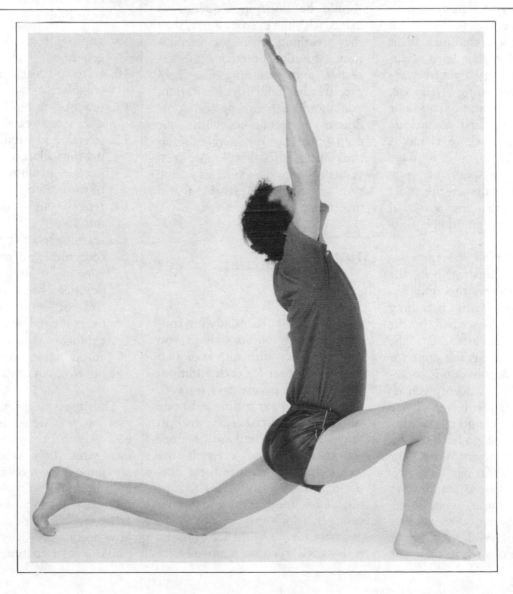

The courses and special routines outlined here are based on our current beginner's curriculum of three consecutive ten-week courses. You may move slightly slower or faster, since each individual has different needs and capacities, but be sure that you don't become so eager to progress that you strain or fail to pay attention to mastering the details of each technique. The Maintenance Routines at the end of each section are designed to keep you in practice indefinitely until you feel like going on to the next course. Asterisks indicate techniques new to that particular week or course.

The best way to start is to read over the entire course to get an idea of how the techniques all fit together. We feel that yoga is approached best as a balanced experience encompassing exercise, breathing and meditation, and our classes are structured to include some of each of these elements each week. Even if you don't have a lot of time to spend on yoga each day, you will get the most benefit from including some of each element in your daily practice session.

You will find all the exercises described and illustrated in the chapter that follows this one, Exercises (Asans), with breathing and meditation described in the two next chapters after that. The warm-up sequence is the same for each course. Warming up is so important that it has been given its own chapter. If you have skipped the previous chapter, Getting Ready to Exercise, go back!

In the chapter on Asans, the yoga exercises proper are presented in order from standing to kneeling to sitting to lying down. We have organized the exercises this way so that you do not have to flip back and forth in the book

as you follow the curriculum. You will notice that each exercise is marked with a Roman numeral—a I, II or III—which stands for the first, second or third course. Advanced exercises are shown along with their simpler versions. *Please do not attempt the more advanced version until the curriculum instructs you to do so.* This will avoid injury or stress by building your strength and stamina safely and properly.

As you follow the course guidelines, remember the importance of making a smooth transition from one exercise to the next. Many students ask if the techniques should be done in sequence as listed, with the exercises first, then the breathing, then the meditation. Although practicing the exercises and breathing first help prepare the mind for meditation, you should experiment and coordinate the techniques with your own schedule. You may split up the routine, also, if it is more convenient, doing the exercises at one time of day, and breathing and meditating at another.

COURSE ONE

Introduction

Remember that the following routines are *suggestions* only. If you find the pace difficult, take two weeks or longer for each addition. If the routine is very easy for you, and you have extra time, add one or two new exercises each week so that you move along a little more quickly. However, even if the asans are easy, practice them during the first month for the recommended amount of time and in the order in which they are given. In each course the sequence of asans is designed so you can move easily

from one to the other, and from standing to kneeling to sitting, and finally to lying down.

The objectives for the first ten weeks of a yoga program are to:

1. strengthen and stretch the spine and legs
2. improve circulation
3. begin to limber the hips and knee joints
4. learn to coordinate the breath with the asans
5. improve kinesthetic sense
6. improve balance and coordination
7. stretch major muscle groups
8. begin to communicate with your body
9. improve respiration and oxygenation
10. learn to breathe correctly and completely
11. practice using breath to reduce stress reactions
12. stretch and strengthen breathing musculature
13. practice extension and control of the breath
14. refresh and recharge your mind
15. learn to relax at will
16. recognize and release muscle tension
17. practice observation and control of sensory input and other mental activities
18. explore detachment from emotional stress reactions
19. improve concentration

The most important goal in the first few weeks is to find the best way to fit your yoga practice into your daily schedule. Don't set impossible goals. Start with a minimum time—even five minutes—that you *know* you can achieve every single day, no matter how hectic your schedule. Practice thinking of odd times during the day when you can fit in a technique or two (see Chapter 10 on stress for ideas). Then any additional time you can put in will be a bonus. You'll feel better about yourself and your practices when you can fulfill your commitment. And that good self-image will motivate you to continue practicing.

NOTE FOR WOMEN:

Following is a modfied routine to practice during your menstrual cycle. If you wish to add any other exercises, refer back to the guidelines in the introductory chapter, p. 17.

Here is your alternate routine of yoga asans. Use your common sense: If you notice unusual cramping, pain or extra-heavy bleeding, stop at once.

Shoulder Roll
Elbow Touch
Arm Roll
Standing Reach
Leg Lifts
Use barre for leg stretches
Tree Pose
Easy Bend
Sit between feet; practice seated
    positions
Arm Reach
Ankle Stretch
Knee/Ankle Massage
Limber Hips
Ankle Rotations and Foot Flaps
Alternate Toe Touch
Laughasan
Leg Raises (lie on side, head on
    elbow)
Hamstring stretch on back (hold
    toes, slowly try to straighten
    leg)

WEEKLY CURRICULUM

(*indicates new exercise)

Week One

ASANS
Warm-up sequence (pp. 21–34)
Easy Balance (p. 54)
Stretching Dog (p. 56)
Alternate Triangle (p. 59)
Corpse Pose Rest (p. 52)
Knee Squeeze (single only) (p. 99)
Foot Flaps (p. 86)
Seated Sun Pose (p. 86)
Baby Pose (p. 53)
Back Strengtheners (single arm
    and alternate arm and leg only)
    (p. 116)

BREATHING
(Breath Warm-ups)
Back Arch (p. 134)
Arm Swing (p. 135)
Arm Reach (p. 135)
Belly Breath (10 repetitions or
    more per day to start) (p. 136)

MEDITATION
10 to 15 minutes, lying down

Week Two

ASANS
Warm-up sequence
Easy Balance
Stretching Dog
Alternate Triangle
*Standing Sun Pose (p. 70)
Corpse Pose Rest
Knee Squeeze (* add double)
    (p. 99)
Foot Flaps
Seated Sun Pose
Baby Pose
Back Strengtheners (* add arms
    only and legs only) (p. 116)

BREATHING
All Breath Warm-ups
*Complete Breath (p. 137)

MEDITATION
10 to 15 minutes

Week Three

ASANS
Warm-up sequence
Easy Balance
Stretching Dog
Alternate Triangle
Standing Sun Pose
Corpse Pose Rest
Knee Squeeze
Foot Flaps
Seated Sun Pose
*Alternate Seated Sun Pose (p. 89)
Baby Pose
Back Strengtheners
*Boat Pose (p. 117)

BREATHING
All Breath Warm-ups
*Lion (p. 139)
Complete Breath—work on
    rhythm and smoothness

MEDITATION
10 to 15 minutes
This week—Body Talk; see
    p. 38.

Week Four

ASANS
Warm-up sequence
Easy Balance
*Easy Balance Twist (p. 55)
*Complete Leg Lift (p. 32)
Stretching Dog
Alternate Triangle
Standing Sun Pose
Corpse Pose Rest
Knee Squeeze
Foot Flaps
Seated Sun Pose
Alternate Seated Sun Pose
Baby Pose
*Easy Cobra Pose (p. 120)
Back Strengtheners
Boat Pose

BREATHING
All Breath Warm-ups
Lion
Complete Breath—start timing
    your breath using clock; (p. 138)
    start using earplugs

MEDITATION
10 to 15 minutes

In about the third week of our curriculum, we insert the following exercise to augment the process of communication with your body. After you have tried the techniques for a couple of weeks and have had a chance to observe how they are affecting you, try this exercise.

BE NICE TO YOUR BODY: BODY TALK

Have you ever noticed how difficult it is to think creatively when you are ill or injured? Or conversely, when you are immersed in an emotional or intellectual problem, do you find yourself not as willing to spend the time to take care of your body in the healthiest way? The mind and body are intimately connected; by affecting one, you automatically affect the other. This is why yoga stresses the importance of attaining and maintaining as high a state of health as possible in all aspects of life.

Try having a conversation with your body to find out more about its needs. Have paper and pen ready. Sit in a comfortable position, close your eyes and for a few minutes think back on your relationship with your body throughout your life. Try to remember as many physical experiences as you can, and make a list of at least eight of these experiences. Try to write down some from childhood, some from adolescence and some current experiences. Some examples: learning to ride a bicycle; running for a touchdown in high school; giving birth.

Now try to remember how you felt about your body at these various stages in your life. For example, everyone goes through dramatic physical changes in early adolescence. Try to remember how you felt about your body—its look, shape and capabilities—during that period of your life. Isn't it true that we tend to take our bodies for granted and focus on the deficiences rather than the assets?

Now just relax, close your eyes and take a few deep breaths. Try to quiet your mind very gently.

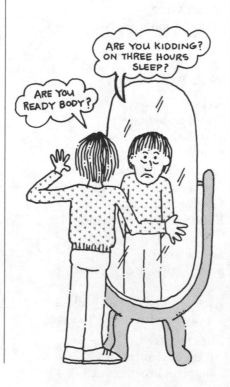

When you feel relaxed, open your eyes and write down a greeting to your body. Imagine that you are standing in front of a mirror and that your body could talk out loud to you. What would it say? Write down whatever comes into your mind. Now close your eyes again, relax, quiet your mind, breathe deeply and wait until your response to what your body has said occurs to you. Write that down. Then close your eyes, relax and wait for your body's response. Write it down. If you have a particular physical problem, ask your body specifically about that problem.

Continue this process for about ten minutes. At the end of that time you should have a brief written conversation that may tell you something about how your body feels and about its needs and desires. Even if you feel you are making up the whole conversation, your imagination is largely fueled by your unconscious, and you may be surprised by what your body "says" to you in this context.

Normally we only listen to our body when it gives us the obvious signals of pain or strain, hunger or thirst or exhaustion. By regularly tuning in to your body with this technique, you will gradually develop a much healthier relationship with it. You'll learn to recognize its warning signals so that you can relax muscle tension before it develops into a headache or stomach upset, give it the kinds of food it most needs. You will also grow to respect the amazing ways your body functions in order to maintain the precious gift of life that allows us to grow and learn.

Week Five

ASANS
Warm-up sequence
Easy Balance
Easy Balance Twist
Complete Leg Lift
Stretching Dog
Alternate Triangle
*Full Triangle (p. 58)
Standing Sun Pose
Corpse Pose Rest
Knee Squeeze
Foot Flaps
Seated Sun Pose
Alternate Seated Sun Pose
Baby Pose
Easy and * Regular Cobra
    (pp. 120, 121)
Back Strengtheners
Boat Pose
*Easy Bridge Rest (p. 104)

BREATHING
All Breath Warm-ups
Lion
Complete Breath—continue
    timing breath

MEDITATION
10 to 15 minutes

Week Six

ASANS
Warm-up sequence
Easy Balance and Twist
Complete Leg Lift
*Tree Pose (p. 64)
Stretching Dog
Alternate Triangle
Standing Sun Pose
Corpse Pose Rest
Knee Squeeze
Foot Flaps
Seated Sun Pose
Alternate Seated Sun Prose
*Limber Hips (p. 90)
Baby Pose
*Easy Spine Twist (p. 91)
Back Strengtheners
Boat Pose
*Rock and Roll (p. 109)
Easy Bridge

BREATHING
All Breath Warm-ups
Lion
Complete Breath
*Humming Breath (p. 138)

MEDITATION
10 to 15 minutes

By this time you have added so many new asans to your repertoire that unless you have an expandable schedule, you won't be able to fit everything in. If that is the case, each day drop out several of the earlier asans, but make them different each day so you still get some practice of each. You may also use the shorter routines on pp. 40 and 41 when time is short.

Week Seven

ASANS
Warm-up sequence
Easy Balance and Twist
Complete Leg Lift
Tree Pose
*Dancer Pose (p. 66)
Stretching Dog
Alternate Triangle
Full Triangle
Standing Sun Pose
Corpse Pose Rest
Knee Squeeze
Foot Flaps
Seated Sun Pose
Alternate Seated Sun Pose
Limber Hips
Baby Pose
*Full Spine Twist (p. 92)
*Diamond Pose (p. 95)
Boat Pose
*Bow Pose (p. 122)
Rock and Roll
Easy Bridge

BREATHING
All Breath Warm-ups
Lion
Complete Breath—continue
    timing breath occasionally
Humming Breath

MEDITATION
10 to 15 minutes

Week Eight

ASANS
Warm-up sequence
Easy Balance and Twist
Complete Leg Lift
Tree Pose
Stretching Dog
Alternate Triangle
Full Triangle
Standing Sun Pose
Corpse Pose Rest
Knee Squeeze
Foot Flaps
Seated Sun Pose
Alternate Seated Sun Pose
Limber Hips
Baby Pose
*Alternate Arm and Leg Balance
    (p. 73)
*Bow Variation (p. 76)
Spine Twist
Bow Pose
Boat Pose
Rock and Roll
*Shoulder Stand (p. 110)
Easy Bridge

BREATHING
All Breath Warm-ups
Lion
Complete Breath—continue
    timing breath occasionally
Humming Breath

MEDITATION
15 to 20 minutes

Week Nine

ASANS
Warm-up sequence
Easy Balance and Twist
Complete Leg Lift
Tree Pose
Dancer Pose
*T Pose (p. 67)
Standing Rest
Stretching Dog
Alternate Triangle
Full Triangle

Standing Sun Pose
Corpse Pose Rest
Knee Squeeze
Foot Flaps
Seated Sun Pose
Alternate Seated Sun Pose
Limber Hips
Baby Pose
Alternate Arm and Leg Balance
Bow Variation
*Cat Breath (p. 74)
Spine Twist
Back Strengtheners
Boat Pose
Rock and Roll
Shoulder Stand
*Pelvic Twist (p. 103)
*Intense Floor Stretch (p. 98)
Easy Bridge

BREATHING
All Breath Warm-ups
Lion
Complete Breath
Humming Breath

MEDITATION
15 to 20 minutes

Week Ten

ASANS
Warm-up sequence
Easy Balance and Twist
Complete Leg Lift
Tree Pose
Dancer Pose
T Pose
Standing Rest
Stretching Dog
Alternate Triangle
Full Triangle
Standing Sun Pose
Corpse Pose Rest
Knee Squeeze
Foot Flaps
Seated Sun Pose
Alternate Seated Sun Pose
Limber Hips
Baby Pose
Alternate Arm and Leg Balance
Bow Variation
Cat Breath
Spine Twist
Back Strengtheners
Boat Pose
Rock and Roll

Shoulder Stand
*Plow Pose (p. 112)
Pelvic Twist
Intense Floor Stretch
Easy Bridge

BREATHING
All Breath Warm-ups
Lion
Complete Breath
Humming Breath

MEDITATION
15 to 20 minutes

Maintenance Routine I

After finishing a course, students sometimes wish to practice on their own for a while before starting another. This routine will keep you in practice until you feel ready to go on. The routine provides essential stretching and strengthening exercises. Some variations are indicated (in parenthesis), also, so you won't get bored. Don't forget breathing and meditation!

ROUTINE
Warm-up sequence
Easy Balance
    (Easy Balance Twist)
Tree Pose
    (Dancer or T Pose)
Standing Rest
Alternate Triangle
    (Full Triangle)
Standing Sun Pose
Baby Pose
Arm and Leg Balance
    (Bow Variation)
Cat Breath
    (Stretching Dog)
Alternate Seated Sun Pose
Spine Twist
    (Pelvic Twist)
Diamond Pose
    (Limber Hips)
Cobra Pose
Bow Pose
    (Boat Pose)
Knee Squeeze
Easy Bridge
Shoulder Stand

FATIGUE-REDUCING ROUTINE

Try this shorter routine on days when you are very tired and have no time for a full asan routine. Asans that compress (such as the knee squeezes) or those that bend backward (such as the Easy Cobra) are the most effective when you are under stress, because they help relax tensed breathing and release tight postural muscles.

Shoulder Roll, p. 21
Elbow Touch, p. 22
Easy Bend, then hang head down for several seconds, p. 27
Easy Balance, p. 54
Baby Pose, p. 53
Cat Breath, p. 74
Easy Cobra, p. 120
Easy Spine Twist, p. 91
Knee Squeeze, p. 99
Easy Bridge, p. 104

Always include at least three Complete Breaths and at least a minute or two of meditation.

COURSE TWO

Introduction

After your first ten weeks of practice, you will have a comprehensive repertoire of asans you are performing smoothly and deliberately, paying attention to details and not straining past your capacity.

You should feel comfortable about moving on to the second course if:

1. You are practicing at least four days per week.
2. Your complete breath cycle is smooth and correct, using the three stages; the length is at least 10 seconds in and 10 seconds out (remember, no holding of breath at top or bottom); and Humming Breath is 3 to 5 seconds in and at least 15 seconds out.
3. You feel comfortable with your relaxation process and practice meditation at least four days per week.
4. You have found a seated position (kneeling, crosslegged or in a chair) you can hold without discomfort for at least 5 minutes.
5. Your performance of asans is smooth and slow, using the proper breath pattern for each pose.

Notice that there is no standard for limberness—the final position you are able to attain without strain at each point in your progress is less important than the position and coordination of your breath and mind.

In this second ten-week course, the objectives are to:

1. Limber hips and knees to improve seated position.
2. Identify breath patterns for each asan.
3. Continue back-strengthening asan work.
4. Learn new breath techniques for stress management, greater quietness and improved oxygenation.
5. Become familiar with the practice of Asan Point.
6. Build a steady practice schedule of at least 15 minutes per day.
7. Experiment with a seated meditation technique.
8. Learn the Sun Salutation (*Surya Namaskar*) asan sequence.

Asan Point

The concept of Asan Point is based on the assumption that asans are ninety percent mental and only ten percent physical. This means that your attention shifts from the physical pose to a state of mind that is similar to meditation: quiet, focused, aware. When you have reached a transition point in an asan—for example, the top of the Cobra pose—you stop for a moment (just a second or two). No extraneous muscle groups are being used; your face is relaxed; you've checked details such as the correct position of fingers and eyes; your breath is either in or out, and is not strained. Finally, your mind becomes poised in stillness. For a two-second period your whole being rests. This is the Asan Point. When you have learned this technique correctly, your exercise routine will bring on a state of mind similar to that of meditation.

Breath Patterns in Asans. You may have noticed already that different asans employ different breath patterns. These are important, because they have to do with why the asans have the effects that they do. Here are some examples of each:

Complete Breath: Simple in/out breaths of even lengths. The Com-

---

SHORT ROUTINE FOR BUSY DAYS

For those times when you are feeling energetic but in a pinch for time, this routine will give you essential stretches and strengtheners. It includes more strenuous asans, such as the Cobra and Shoulder Stand, so you must do a full warm-up sequence first.

Warm-ups, pp. 20-34
Alternate Triangle, p. 59
T Pose, p. 67
Standing Sun Pose, p. 70
Baby Pose, p. 164
Arm and Leg Balance, p. 73
Alternate Seated Sun Pose, p. 89
Pelvic Twist, p. 103
Cobra Pose, p. 121
Shoulder Stand, p. 110

End with at least three Complete Breaths and at least a minute or two of meditation.

NOTE FOR WOMEN:

It is even more important now to follow our suggestion about not practicing difficult asans during your menstrual period. The asans and breathing you will be learning in this course are more strenuous, and your mind and emotions will become much more sensitive. Substitute the routine outlined on p. 37, or try this alternative: twenty minutes of other exercise, such as walking, swimming, bicycling; twenty-minute nap; twenty-minute study of yoga or related texts (see Bibliography for suggestions).

---

plete Breath pattern allows the greatest volume of air to be inhaled and exhaled.

Examples: Full Bend, Cobra V-Raise, Alternate Arm and Leg Balance, Cat Breath.

Exterior Hold: Short hold at bottom of exhalation. This extra hold allows more waste products to be exhaled, so this breath pattern is often called a purifying breath.

Examples: Standing and Seated Sun Pose, Alternate Triangle.

Interior Hold: Short hold at top of inhalation. Briefly holding an inhalation allows more oxygen to be absorbed into the bloodstream.

Examples: Cobra Pose, Bow Pose, Boat Pose.

Interior Compressed Hold: Short hold at top of inhalation with compression of midsection. This pattern intensifies the action of the Interior Hold.

Examples: Easy Balance and Twist, Knee Squeeze.

Easy Breath: A completely non-manipulated breath pattern, when the breathing muscles are relaxed. In the following examples of very different types of exercises, the rate or intensity of the breath may change, but the breathing muscles will still be relaxed. The Easy Breath allows the body to choose its own rhythm of breathing as

you relax your body in a holding pose.

Examples: Balance poses such as the Dancer Pose, Tree Pose, and T Pose; other holding poses such as the Pigeon Hold, the Spine Twist and the Baby Pose.

As an experiment, do your warm-up sequence as usual but, instead of going on to your regular asan routine, try each of the asans just listed and see if you can observe how the breath changes in each one. Remember to pay attention to details such as the position of your fingers and toes, and make sure that only the required muscle groups for each asan are employed.

WEEKLY CURRICULUM

(*indicates new exercise)

Week One

ASANS
Warm-up sequence, adding *Hip Rock (p. 57), *Hip Rotation (p. 56), *Side Triangle (p. 60) after Full Bends
Tree Pose
Dancer Pose
Standing Sun Pose
Alternate Arm and Leg Balance
Cat Breath
*Thigh Stretch (p. 172)
Corpse Pose Rest
*Easy Fish Pose (p. 102)
Baby Pose
Back Strengtheners
Knee Squeeze
Easy Bridge
Shoulder Stand
Plow Pose

BREATHING
Breath Warm-Ups
Lion
Complete Breath—if length is not up to 10 seconds in, 10 seconds out, practice breath extension before moving on to next breath technique
*Kapalabhati—10 seconds bellows; three complete cycles (p. 141)

MEDITATION
15 to 20 minutes, lying down

Week Two

ASANS
Warm-up sequence
*Twisting Triangle (p. 61)
Tree Pose
Dancer Pose
*T Pose Knee Bends (p. 69)
Standing Sun Pose
*Cobra V-Raise (p. 77)
Baby Pose
Alternate Arm and Leg Balance
Cat Breath

Thigh Stretch
Corpse Pose Rest
Fish Pose
Baby Pose
Back Strengtheners
Knee Squeeze
Easy Bridge
Shoulder Stand
Plow Pose
Alternatively, this week practice identifying breath patterns in the different asans (see introduction to Course Two).

BREATHING
Breath Warm-ups
Lion
*Bramari Breath (p. 142)
Complete Breath—5 cycles
Kapalabhati—10 seconds bellows; three complete cycles. Work on evenness of movement and sound.

MEDITATION
15 to 20 minutes. Start practicing seated position for meditation. (See section on posture in Breathing chapter.) Concentrate on achieving a fully relaxed body and a stable position. Hold until you start feeling discomfort, then finish meditation lying down.

Week Three

ASANS
Warm-up sequence
Twisting Triangle
Dancer Pose
Standing Sun Pose
Cobra V-Raise
Alternate Arm and Leg Balance
Cat Breath
Thigh Stretch
Corpse Pose Rest
Fish Pose
*Ankle Stretch (p. 81)
Baby Pose
Knee Squeeze
Easy Bridge
Shoulder Stand
*Sun Salutation (p. 123)

BREATHING
Breath Warm-ups
Lion
*Laughasan (p. 140)
Complete Breath—5 cycles
Bramari Breath
Kapalabhati—20 seconds bellows; three complete cycles

MEDITATION
15 to 20 minutes, lying down

Week Four

ASANS
Warm-up sequence
Tree Pose
Dancer Pose
T Pose Knee Bends
Standing Sun Pose
Alternate Arm and Leg Balance
Bow Variation
*Camel (p. 82)
Thigh Stretch
Corpse Pose Rest
Fish Pose
Ankle Stretch
Baby Pose
*Pigeon Pose and Hold (p. 84)
Back Strengtheners
Knee Squeeze
Easy Bridge
Shoulder Stand
Plow Pose
Sun Salutation

BREATHING
Breath Warm-Ups
Lion
Bramari Breath
Kapalabhati—20 seconds bellows, faster speed; three complete cycles

MEDITATION
15 to 20 minutes—try seated meditation this week

Week Five

ASANS
Warm-up sequence
Tree Pose
Dancer Pose
T Pose Knee Bends

Standing Sun Pose
Alternate Arm and Leg Balance
Bow Variation
Camel
Thigh Stretch
Corpse Pose Rest
Fish Pose
Baby Pose
*Hero Pose Variation (p. 79)
*Extended Hero Pose (p. 80)
Pigeon Pose and Hold
Back Strengtheners
Knee Squeeze
*Neck Curls (p. 106)
Easy Bridge
Shoulder Stand
Plow Pose
Sun Salutation

BREATHING
Breath warm-ups
Lion
Bramari Breath
Kapalabhati—20 seconds bellows, faster speed; three complete cycles

MEDITATION
15 to 20 minutes, lying down

Week Six

ASANS
Warm-up sequence
Tree Pose
Dancer Pose
T Pose Knee Bends
Standing Sun Pose
Alternate Arm and Leg Balance
Cat Breath
Camel
Thigh Stretch
Corpse Pose Rest
Fish Pose
Ankle Stretch
Baby Pose
Hero Variation
Extended Hero Pose
Pigeon Pose and Hold
Back Strengtheners
Knee Squeeze
Neck Curl
*Easy Sit-Up (p. 105)
*Sun Balance (p. 88)

Easy Bridge
Shoulder Stand
*Plow Variations (p. 112)
Sun Salutation

BREATHING

*Neti (p. 140)
Breath warm-ups
Lion
Bramari Breath
Kapalabhati—20 seconds bellows, faster speed; three complete cycles

MEDITATION

15 to 20 minutes—try seated meditation again this week

Week Seven

ASANS

Warm-up sequence
*Windmill (p. 62)
Tree Pose
Dancer Pose
T Pose Knee Bends
Standing Sun Pose
Alternate Arm and Leg Balance
Cat Breath
Camel
Thigh Stretch
Corpse Pose Rest
Fish Pose
Baby Pose
Spine Twist
Diamond Pose
*Hero Pose (p. 96)
Pigeon Pose and Hold
Back Strengtheners
Knee Squeeze
Neck Curl
Sun Balance
Easy Bridge
Shoulder Stand
Plow Pose

BREATHING

Neti
Breath warm-ups
Lion
Bramari Breath
Complete Breath—5 cycles
Kapalabhati—20 seconds bellows, faster speed; five complete cycles

MEDITATION

15 to 20 minutes—try seated meditation this week

Week Eight

ASANS

Warm-up sequence
Windmills
Tree Pose
Dancer Pose
T Pose Knee Bends
Standing Sun Pose
Alternate Arm and Leg Balance
Cat Breath
Camel
Thigh Stretch
Corpse Pose Rest
Fish Pose
Baby Pose
Hero Pose
Pigeon Pose and Hold
Back Strengtheners
Knee Squeeze
Neck Curl
*Big Sit-up (p. 107)
Easy Bridge
*Alternate Toe Touch (p. 101)
*Walk (p. 100)
Shoulder Stand
Plow Pose

BREATHING

Breath Warm-ups
Lion
Bramari Breath
Kapalabhati—20 seconds bellows, faster speed; five complete cycles

MEDITATION

15 to 20 minutes, lying down or seated

Week Nine

ASANS

Warm-up sequence
Windmills
Tree Pose
Dancer Pose
T Pose Knee Bends
Standing Sun Pose
Alternate Arm and Leg Balance
Cat Breath

Camel
Thigh Stretch
Corpse Pose Rest
Fish Pose
Baby Pose
Hero Pose
Pigeon Pose and Hold
*Airplane Series (p. 118)
Knee Squeeze
Neck Curl
Big Sit-up
*Easy Bridge with Hold (p. 104)
Alternate Toe Touch
Walk
Shoulder Stand
Plow Pose

BREATHING

Breath Warm-ups
Lion
Complete Breath
Bramari Breath
Kapalabhati—30 seconds bellows, maintain speed; five complete cycles

MEDITATION

15 to 20 minutes, seated meditation for at least 5 minutes, the rest of the times lying down

Week Ten

ASANS

Warm-up sequence
Windmills
Tree Pose
Dancer Pose
T Pose Knee Bends
Standing Sun Pose
Alternate Arm and Leg Balance
Cat Breath
Camel
Thigh Stretch
Corpse Pose Rest
Fish Pose
Baby Pose
Pigeon Pose and Hold
Cobra Pose
Airplane Series
Knee Squeeze
Neck Curl
Big Sit-up

Easy Bridge with Hold
Alternate Toe Touch
Shoulder Stand
Plow Pose
Sun Salutation

BREATHING

Breath Warm-ups
Lion
Complete Breath
Bramari Breath
Kapalabhati—30 seconds bellows,
   faster speed; five complete
   cycles

MEDITATION

15 to 20 minutes, seated at least 5
   minutes, lying down for
   remainder.

Maintenance Routine II

Below left, is a maintenance routine for keeping you in practice after the second course. Alternate it with the routine on the right, which is shorter but includes the more strenuous Sun Salutation.

Warm-up Sequence	Warm-Up Sequence
Windmills	Windmills
T Pose and Knee Bends	Dancer Pose
Standing Sun Pose	Cobra V-raise
Cobra V-raise	Thigh stretch
Baby Pose	Baby Pose
Extended Hero Pose	Sun Salutation
Pigeon and Hold	Rest in Corpse Pose
Spine Twist	Knee Squeeze
Seated Sun Pose	Shoulder Stand
Diamond Pose	
Cobra Pose	
Airplane Series	
Neck Curls	
Shoulder Stand	

COURSE THREE

Introduction

If you have been following the curriculum already outlined, you will have been practicing for nearly four months now. In this third stage of practice you will continue more intensely the format introduced with the Sun Salutation in the previous course, with special emphasis on a routine we call the Emotional Stability Routine.

The objectives of this course are to:

1. Learn to recognize the target zones for retention of muscle tension in your body.
2. Strengthen stomach and back muscles.
3. Increase stamina.
4. Improve stress resistance.
5. Learn to recognize and release tight breathing patterns.

To understand how the Emotional Stability Routine works, we have to talk about stress. Unlike other living beings, which experience a stress reaction and then go back to normal, humans often retain the tension or upset (physical or mental) because our memory and self-awareness gives us the capacity to replay a stressful event again and again in our minds and every time we replay it, the deeper it is etched in our memory. It's as if we have had in our heads a cassette library of old, unresolved business.

When we replay that kind of memory, our bodies reexperience their original responses to it: pulse and breathing speed up, blood pressure increases and hormone messengers are activated. Although our body does more or less return to a normal state after one of these episodes, it is so deluged by the constant demand for readiness and response that it often retains muscle tension and other stress responses longer than normal—in many cases almost constantly.

Obviously, as this residual tension accumulates, we feel stiffer and more physically tense. Circulation may be constricted in the head because of tight neck muscles, and we may experience increasing fatigue, lethargy, headaches and a reduced ability to cope. Emotions become jangled and more out of control—physical constriction produces mental constriction.

The Emotional Stability Routine counters this syndrome with a routine based on the theory that if physical constriction produces emotional constriction, then physical strength and release produce emotional strength and release. A group of techniques that act to release physical constriction (and therefore emotional tension) in target areas, the Emotional Stability Routine strengthens stress-vulnerable zones of the body and makes them more resilient to the stress inflicted on them by stressful experiences or memories of those experiences.

The target zones for the Emotional Stability Routine are (in order of most common tension, pain or other negative stress response): the stomach, breath, face, upper back and neck, knees, thighs, lower back, throat and ankles. Emotional blocks and frustrations seem to move throughout the body, lodging in successive areas and causing stiffness, pain, fear, anxiety or other tension-related symptoms. The Emotional Stability Routine physically strengthens these vulnerable body parts, building resistance to attack from the emotions.

The Emotional Stability Routine works best when it is practiced every day for the first month, then about two to three times per week. Daily practice in the beginning helps establish solidly the beneficial effects. However, you will notice that the Emotional Stability Routine does not include several classes of asans—for example, those that work on limberness of hips and knees and those that stretch the front of the thighs and the back of the legs. On the three or four days that you don't practice the Emotional Stability Routine, practice an alternate routine (see example, p. 47) that compensates for these deficits.

An easier version of the Emotional Stability Routine is given at the beginning of this chapter. Practice it for at least two weeks; then go on to the second version, which adds repetitions and some new exercises. Finally, after at least four weeks of practice, you can start the full routine. By the end of six weeks, you should evaluate the effects of the routine using the Body Talk exercise as described earlier in this chapter (p. 38). Talk to different parts of your body individually, especially the target zones of the Emotional Stability Routine.

WEEKLY CURRICULUM

It is important to remember that to be most effective, the Emotional Stability Routine should be considered not just an asan routine but a sequence of asans, breathing and meditation.

EMOTIONAL STABILITY ROUTINE, VERSION I

Weeks One and Two

ASANS
Warm-up Sequence
leave out the Hands and Knees Stretch, since it is included later in the main body of asans in this routine)
Windmills (3 each side)
Cobra V-raise (3)
*Forward Plank (1 each side) (p. 78)
Baby Pose (until breath returns to normal)
*Hands and Knees Stretch—with double breath (3) (p. 34)
Cat Breath (3)
Arm and Leg Balance (3 each side)
*Easy Plow Breath (3) (p. 114)
Neck Curls (3)
Alternate Toe Touch (3 each side)
*Side Stretch (1 each side, then reverse feet and repeat) (p. 97)
*Spinal Arch (3) (p. 143)

BREATHING
Complete Breath—five cycles
Kapalabhati—30 seconds bellows; five cycles

MEDITATION
5 minutes at least seated, remainder lying down

EMOTIONAL STABILITY ROUTINE, VERSION II

Weeks Three and Four

ASANS
Warm-up sequence
Windmills (3 to 6 each side)
Cobra V-raise (3 to 6)
Forward plank
*Side Plank (p. 78)
Baby Pose (at least 1 minute, or until breath returns to normal)
Hands and Knees Stretch with double breath
*Cat Breath Variation (p. 75)
Easy Plow Breath (3 to 6)
Walk
Neck Curls
Big Sit-up (instead of, or in addition to, Neck Curls)
Alternate Toe Touch
Side Stretch
Spinal Arch

BREATHING
Complete Breath—five cycles
Kapalabhati—five cycles

MEDITATION
At least 5 minutes seated; total at least 15 minutes

Weeks Five and Six

Now, if you have no physical problems with your back, you may begin the full Emotional Stability Routine, alternating with the routine below it, which provides benefits missed by the routine.

EMOTIONAL STABILITY ROUTINE
Warm-up Sequence
Windmills (6 each side)

Special Note: The Emotional Stability Routine contains strenuous movements that may aggravate a back or neck condition. Do not practice this routine if you have, or suspect you may have, a problem with your spine. If you are not sure, ask your physician for advice. If you start practicing the routine and notice pain in any part of your back, dizziness, headaches or other unusual symptoms, stop the routine immediately and see your physician.

If you have a back problem, and you have your doctor's approval to practice yoga but are not sure how to proceed without doing the Emotional Stability Routine, please write to us for suggestions.

Cobra V-raise (6)
Forward Plank (1)
Side Plank (1)
Baby Pose (1 minute)
Plow Breath or Easy Version (6)
Big Sit-up (6)
Corpse Pose Rest
*Alternate Big Sit-up (6 each side)
   (p. 108)
Side Stretch (2 each foot position)
Spinal Arch (3)

ALTERNATE ROUTINE
Warm-up Sequence
Twisting Triangle
Dancer Pose
T Pose with Knee Bends
Standing Sun Pose or Sun Pose
   Variation
Corpse Pose Rest
Knee Squeeze
Alternate Seated Sun Pose
Limber Hips
Spine Twist
Diamond Pose
Hero Pose
Extended Hero
Baby Pose
Thigh Stretch
Cat Breath
Pigeon and Hold
Cobra Pose
Shoulder Stand
Easy Bridge

BREATHING
Kapalabhati—five cycles; *45
   seconds bellows
 *Agni Kriya (p. 144)

MEDITATION
Seated Meditation at least 10
   minutes

Week Seven

Earlier we talked about how the Emotional Stability Routine is meant to affect those areas of the body—the "target zones"—that respond to stress most often by holding or tightening the breath and other muscles. This week, at least once, go back to the Body Talk exercise (see p. 38) and have a written dialogue with your body, concentrating on particular areas. Try to talk to specific parts, and then talk to your body as a whole, figuring out what physical and emotional effects the routine has brought about.

Start by talking to your *breath*. What physical changes have occurred since you began practicing this routine? Have you noticed any changes in the way your breath responds to stress? Now talk to your *stomach*. How does it feel? Are its muscles any stronger than before? Does it feel more resilient to tension? Does it get upset as often? What is your stomach's attitude toward what you are doing? Now talk to your *face*. How has your face responded to the physical and emotional effects of this routine? When you look in the mirror, does your face look different? How? Does it feel more in control of its muscular reactions? Does it feel any more relaxed? Move on to your *neck and throat*. Does your throat constrict when tense? Any less so since beginning this routine? Are you feeling better able to express your thoughts and feelings? Now move to your *lower back* and talk to that part of your body. Does your lower back feel stronger? Does it feel any more limber? If you have had chronic pain or stiffness in your back, has that improved at all? Does your lower back feel more comfortable when you sit for meditation? Move along to your *hips and thighs*. Are they feeling stronger? More limber? Do you feel freer when you walk or run? If you have been bothered with cramping in your legs, has that improved? Talk to your *knees*. Do they feel stronger? Better able to support you? Are you free from mysterious aches and pains in your knees? Do they complain as much when you are in a seated position for meditation or breathing? Finally, talk to your *ankles*. Do they feel stronger and more supportive? Do they bother you when seated cross-legged?

Talk to your body as a whole. How has it learned to adapt to stress conditions? Has it learned better responses than before? Does it recover faster from stress events? Do you sleep better? Is your metabolism functioning normally? Do you have enough energy to do what you want to do? How is your posture? Does your body have any complaints about the food you are feeding it? About the kinds of activities you do in addition to yoga? About yoga practice? What does your body like most about the Emotional Stability Routine? Least? How can you and your body work together to get the most out of this routine? Continue working on the alternate routines as before.

Week Eight

This week experiment doing the routines at two different speeds. Asan sequences in yoga can be practiced quickly, with shorter, more intense breathing patterns, or more slowly, with longer breath cycles and brief holds at each Asan Point. The faster version of the Emotional Stability Routine, which takes seven to ten minutes, has the advantage of causing your breath to change rapidly; thus your mood can be shifted more easily. The slower version (which takes about 20 minutes) reinforces a concentrated state of mind and attention to the transition points.

When you are practicing the routine at the faster speed, be sure not to get careless about details such as the position of hands and feet, and breathe *as much air* in and out as before, even though you are breathing a little faster. In the slower version, take care not to hold your breath so long at the transition points that you gasp for air. Remember that the full routine includes breathing and meditation as well as the asans.

Week Nine

This week vary your alternate routine to include many asans that you haven't practiced in a while. Include the Sun Salutation especially, and practice this routine in both faster and slower versions if you can. Experiment with creating several other alternate routines for yourself, trying to achieve a balance of stretches and strengtheners.

Week Ten

This week do the Body Talk exercise again, asking the same questions of the different parts of your body (and any new questions that occur to you). See if there has been any change from the last time you did the exercise.

Experiment with the following routine in order to practice holding yoga asans for an extended period of time. Do not practice this routine more than two days in a row. When the routine instructs you to hold a position in which you usually hold the breath in or out, instead let your breath come naturally and relaxed for the holding period (except if you are instructed not to release the breath); however, as you come out of the hold, return to the normal breath pattern to finish the exercise. For example, if you are holding the Seated Sun Pose at the bottom, when your breath is normally held out, release the breath and just relax into the pose. You may have to grasp your legs a bit higher to avoid strain during the hold.

When you are ready to come out of the hold, breathe in as you raise your arms up in a circle overhead, then breathe out and lower your arms to your sides. When holding, adjust the position of your head, if necessary, to prevent strain to your neck.

Do not strain. If the suggested holding intervals make you shaky or fatigued, or cause muscle pain, reduce the length of each. Balance poses are especially revealing of strain; a shaking body should indicate to you that your nervous system has had enough! The length of time that you can hold a position will vary from day to day, depending on your stress levels, fatigue, nutrition, emotions and other factors, so don't be discouraged if you cannot hold a position as long as the day before. Don't strain. Each day's effort—even if it's shorter than the previous day —will contribute to a steady increase in the strength of your nervous system. Remember that the idea is to achieve a relaxed stretch, using only the muscle groups needed for the exercise; keeping the breath pattern smooth and relaxed and the mind poised and still.

Routine for Practicing Holding Positions

Warm-up Sequence	Regular speed
Alternate Triangle	Hold each leg at the bottom stretch for 15 seconds. Release breath while holding.
Standing Rest	Thirty seconds to 1 minute.
Dancer Pose	Hold each side for 30 seconds. Be sure to relax the stomach muscles. Release breath while holding.
Standing Sun Pose	Regular speed
Baby Pose	Thirty seconds to 1 minute.
Cobra V-raise	Hold each transition (extreme up and extreme down) for 3 seconds. Do not release breath.
Baby Pose	Thirty seconds to 1 minute.
Pigeon Pose and Hold	Hold should be 30 seconds. Release breath while holding.
Cat Breath	Hold each extreme position 3 seconds. Do not release breath.
Arm and Leg Balance	Hold alternate arm and leg up for 10 seconds. Release breath while holding.
Easy Cobra	Regular speed
Alternate Seated Sun Pose	Hold downward position 15 seconds. Release breath while holding.
Shoulder Stand.	Hold 30 to 60 seconds.

AFTER COURSE THREE...

If you have been following the courses outlined in this chapter, you have now been practicing yoga for at least seven months. You know over 70 asans, plus several breathing techniques and relaxation and meditation. How do you choose which techniques to practice each day?

You have already learned several routines throughout this curriculum: the Maintenance Routines, the Emotional Stability Routine, among others. You may choose from any of these—or from any of the weekly routines for any course—to add variety to your daily practice. You may also create your own routines. In the back of this book you will find the techniques listed in groups according to their functions (many techniques are listed more than once.) Use this section to create a special routine for yourself that addresses your needs. For example, you may need to strengthen a weak lower back; choose exercises such as the Arm and Leg Balance and the Back Strengtheners. If you have occasional "blue" days, try some of the techniques listed as pertaining to depression. Be sure always to include some exercise, some breathing and some meditation for a well-balanced daily practice.

If you have questions about your personal curriculum, please write to us, and we'll try our best to help you continue your yoga practice in the most productive way.

CHAPTER 4
EXERCISE
(ASANA)

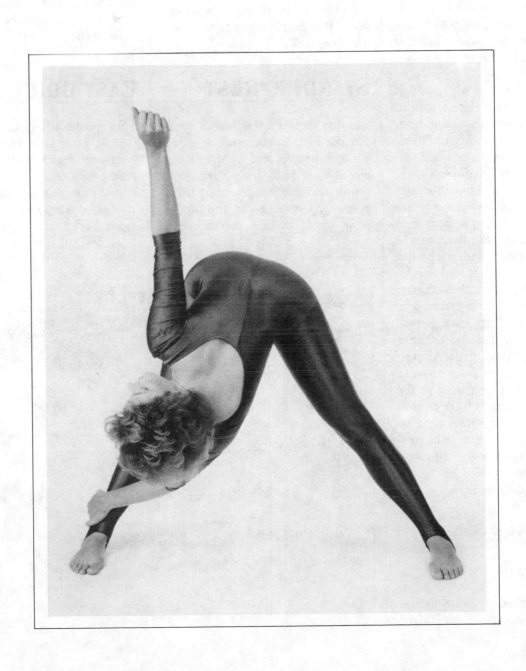

This chapter illustrates and describes each asan listed in the course curricula, and lists the benefits of each. Before you attempt any asans, be sure you have warmed up by following the sequence in Chapter 2, Getting Ready to Exercise. The asans are organized from standing to kneeling, then sitting and lying down. More advanced asans and variations are placed after the easier versions. You will notice a Roman numeral I, II or III next to the title of each asan; this refers to the course curriculum in which the asans first appear. Some asans will be repeated in more than one course.

Remember to read through each exercise first, before trying it. If you have a physical limitation, you may need to modify the exercise in order to perform it comfortably. Remember to move slowly and deliberately, and not to strain. The benefit from doing asans lies not only in achieving a more limber body but in coordinating the physical movement with the breath pattern and a concentrated mind.

As you follow the course curricula, go at your own pace. The weekly routines are suggestions only. If you are elderly, or have physical limitations, proceed even more slowly than usual to give your body time to get used to the movements. You may have to simplify the positions somewhat. Be creative. Yoga is not a rigid process but a fluid one, allowing every individual to find his or her proper pace and intensity.

REST POSES

Relax entire body

After every three or four asans, practicing a rest pose for thirty seconds to one minute will allow your muscles to relax and your breath to return to normal. Use one of the following four positions: Standing Rest, Corpse Pose Rest, Easy Bridge Rest or Baby Pose.

Hold a rest position for 30 to 60 seconds or more, until your breath returns to normal and your muscles relax completely. Close your eyes and quickly check your body's most troublesome tension spots: eyes, jaw, stomach and so on. Let yourself go completely limp. If it helps, imagine that you are a rag doll.

STANDING REST

Stand with feet a few inches apart but parallel. Relax arms at sides. Close your eyes and try to balance equally on both feet. Keep your spine straight; imagine that there is a string attached to the top of your head, pulling you upright.

Pay extra attention to your facial muscles, your shoulders and your stomach, trying to relax as much as possible (A).

CORPSE POSE REST
(Shavasan)

Lie down on your mat, arms at sides or slightly out from your body, with palms facing up. With eyes closed, relax your face, your shoulders, your stomach and any other areas of your body that hold tension (B).

EASY BRIDGE REST

This position is similar to the Corpse Pose Rest but with knees bent and feet flat on the floor a foot or more apart, so that your knees will touch and relax (C). This pose takes more strain off the lower back.

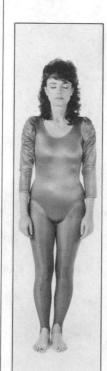

A

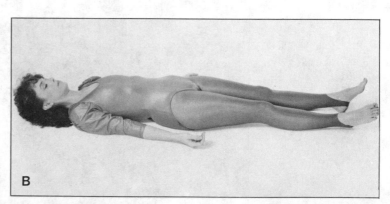

B

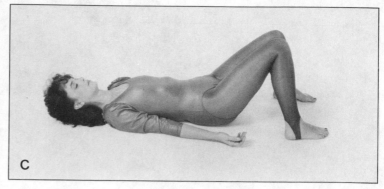

C

BABY POSE

Limbers lower back
Reduces body fat from sides and hips
Improves circulation in pelvic region
Improves digestion
Strengthens knees and ankles
Relieves stiffness in hips, knees and ankles
Improves functioning of the reproductive system

For some of you who are very stiff, this exercise may not be restful at first, so use another rest position to relax and use this as a regular exercise in your routine. Do not do this exercise if you have high blood pressure; instead, sit against the wall to rest.

Sit on your heels with toes flat (D). Bend forward until your head touches the floor. If that is comfortable, bend your arms back, elbows out to the sides, so that your neck and shoulders can relax (E). Your elbows should be resting on the floor. Your head can rest on the floor on your forehead, the bridge of your nose or the top of your head—whatever is comfortable. However, your neck should be straight, so don't turn your head to the side. Breathe normally and relax as much as possible. Wiggle around and find the most comfortable position.

If putting your head on the floor creates too much abdominal discomfort, try one or more of these variations: (1) separate your knees several inches to a foot; (2) cross arms in front of your knees and rest your head on your arms (F); (3) cross your arms on your knees and just bend head forward, being sure to relax the back of the neck.

If your hips or knees are too stiff for this position, try a variation of this exercise called the Folded Pose, using a chair (see p. 179). Sit with your hips against the back of the chair, feet flat, knees slightly apart. Bend forward and let your arms relax over your ankles. (Arms may also be crossed on knees if you experience discomfort due to abdominal compression.) Be sure to relax your neck completely.

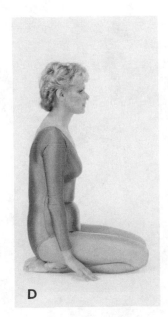

D

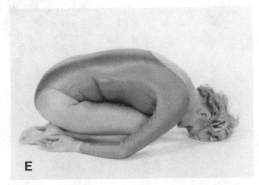

E

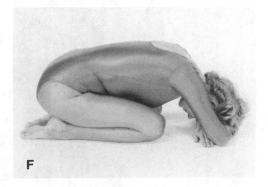

F

EASY BALANCE I

Improves circulation and respiration

Tones the central nervous system

Improves balance and concentration

Strengthens leg muscles, calves and ankles

Helps relieve sciatica and leg cramps

Stand with arms at your sides and exhale (A). Now start to inhale, bringing your arms out slightly and rising up on your toes. Fix your gaze on one spot to help you balance. Complete your inhalation, making sure that you have filled your lungs all the way. Make fists and press them into your diaphragm—just below your rib cage—while holding your breath in (B). Hold for just a second. Then relax, breathe out and come back down on your heels, arms relaxed at sides. Concentrate on a fluidity of movement as you do multiple repetitions. Repetitions: 3 to 5.

- Stare at one spot for balance.
- Make fists just under rib cage.
- Lift and lower heels slowly.

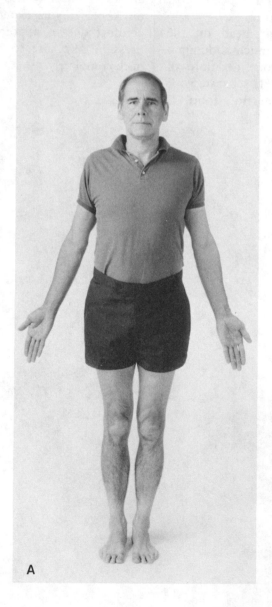

A

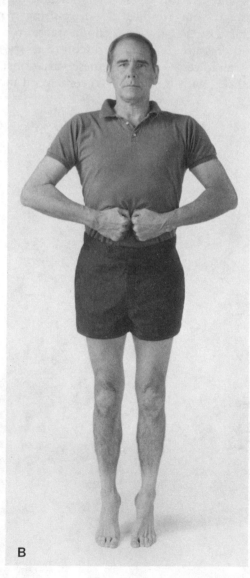

B

EASY BALANCE TWIST I

Improves circulation
Expands chest and lungs
Develops steadiness and poise
Strengthens calves, ankles and toes

Stand with arms at sides. Breathe out. Now breathe in as you rise up on your toes, bringing your arms in a wide circle to the sides and up overhead. Press palms together (A). Steady yourself by fixing your gaze on one spot. Hold your breath in and twist to the right, finding another spot to hold your gaze (B). Twist with your whole body, not just your torso. Then start to breathe out as you turn back to the front, bring your arms back down to the sides in a circle and relax. Repetitions: 3 to each side, alternating.

If you find it difficult to keep your balance as you twist, lower your heels as many times as needed and go back up wherever you are in the exercise sequence.

- Breathe fully and deeply through your nose.
- Stare at one spot for balance.
- Press palms together overhead.
- Twist your whole body, not just your torso.

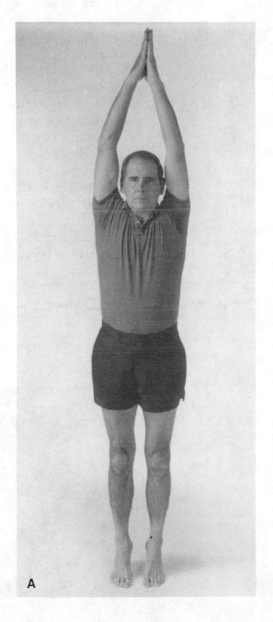

A

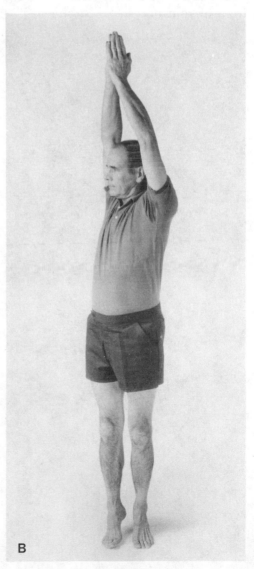

B

STRETCHING DOG I
(Adho Mukhasvanasan)

Limbers shoulder joints, hip joints and tendons in the lower leg
Helps relieve arthritic pain and stiffness in shoulders
Relieves fatigue
Stretches the back of the legs and spine
Increases circulation to the head, rejuvenating brain cells and eyes
Relieves stress on heart muscles, helping with hypertension

Sit on your heels with toes tucked under, hands placed on the floor a few inches in front of your knees. Breathe in and look up, creating a very slight arch in your back (A). Now breathe out and push up into a V, straightening your legs as much as possible and pushing your heels down toward the floor (B). Be careful not to strain! Tuck your head. Now breathe in and lower back into the starting position. Repetitions: 3 to 5.

- Breathe deeply through your nose.
- Tuck your head.
- Try to straighten legs without strain.

HIP ROTATION II, III

Limbers the hip joints, lower back and upper thighs

In Courses II and III add this to the warm-up sequence after the Full Bends. Separate your feet a comfortable distance, but keep your toes pointed forward or slightly inward at all times. Place your hands on your hips, thumbs hooked forward over your hip bone and fingers spread over the lower back for support. (This support will help prevent possible injury from bending backward too far.)

Slowly rotate your hips 360 degrees several times in each direction. Try to stretch the upper thighs and hips as much as possible without strain.

- Keep torso straight.
- Keep feet parallel, toes pointed straight forward or slightly inward.
- Breathe normally.
- Support lower back.

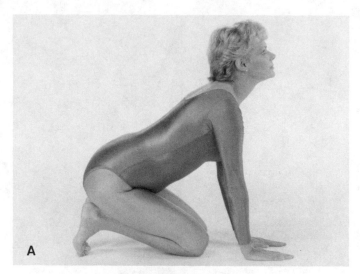

A

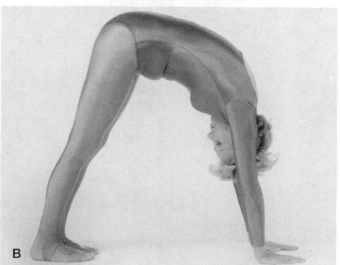

B

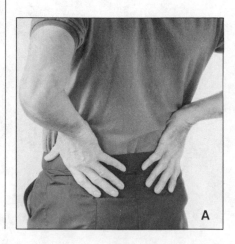

A

HIP ROCK II, III

Limbers hip joints and lower back
Stretches back of the legs
Strengthens lower back
Massages digestive organs
Relieves tension in back and neck

In Courses II and III add this exercise to the warm-up sequence after the Hip Rotation. Starting in the same position as the Hip Rotation (A), breathe in and push hips forward slightly (B), keeping head straight (do *not* drop head back), then breathe out and bend forward, letting arms drop to the floor or as far forward as possible (C). Relax head, neck, arms and back completely. Now breathe in and come back up, replacing hands on hips and pushing forward. Repeat this pumping motion in coordination with the breath. Repetitions: 3 to 5.

- Move slowly and deliberately.
- Breathe fully, through nose.
- Support lower back.
- Keep toes pointed forward or slightly inward.

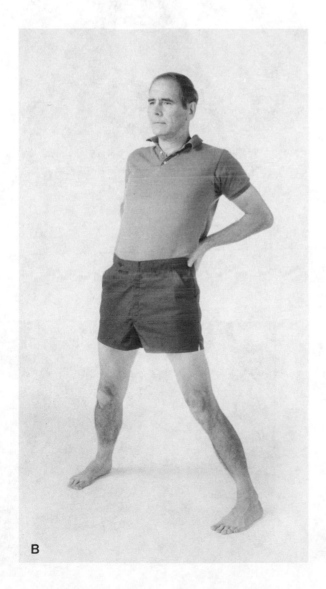

B

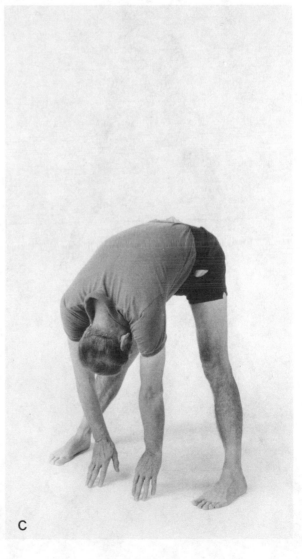

C

FULL TRIANGLE I

(Prasarita Padottanasan)

Limbers and strengthens hamstrings and abductor muscles

Improves circulation and functioning of the kidneys, spleen, stomach, intestines, heart and lungs

Brings fresh blood to head, rejuvenating brain cells

Standing with feet apart, toes pointed in, breathe in and open your arms to the sides (A). Breathe out as you bend forward (B), then grasp both ankles or calves with your hands and finish your exhalation as you pull gently and hold for a moment (C). Then release, cross your arms and hang gently, breathing normally, for a few seconds; eventually you will become so limber that you can rest your crossed arms on the floor (D). Repetitions: 1.

- Breathe normally.
- Keep toes pointed in.

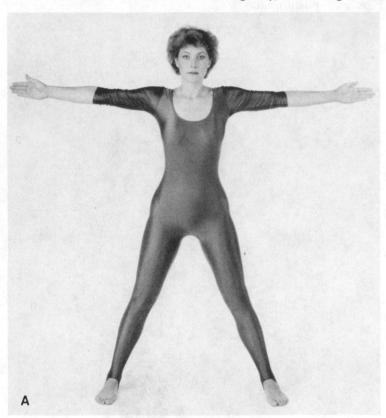

A

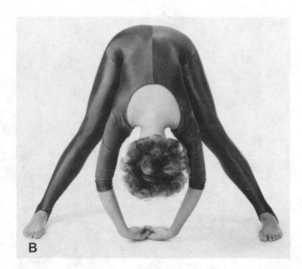

B

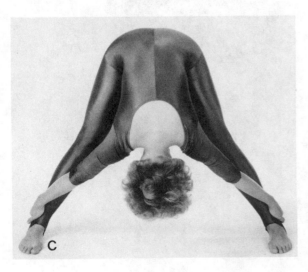

C

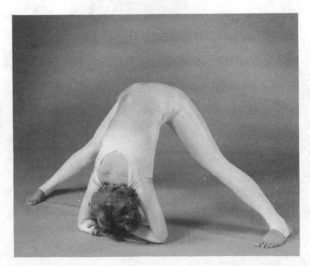

D

ALTERNATE TRIANGLE I

(Trikona Hasthasan)

Localizes and stretches ligaments and nerves in the legs, back and neck

Improves circulation in the entire pelvic region

Reduces body fat in waist

Exercises the intestines and kidneys

Improves circulation to face and eyes

Separate your feet a comfortable distance, with toes pointed forward or slightly inward. To warm up, bend forward gently, first to the center, then to each leg, to be sure that you will not be straining your back. Slowly straighten up.

Breathe in and stretch arms wide, parallel to the floor (A). Now breathe out and slowly bend down to your left leg (E). Grasp the leg with both hands, bend your elbows, keeping your arms close to your body, and gently pull your upper body toward your leg. Your breath should be held completely out. (If you can't bend your elbows, grasp your legs a little higher up. The idea is to pull the upper body by using the arms rather than by using your stomach or lower back muscles, which might cause strain.) Then breathe in and slowly return to a standing position with arms outstretched, and repeat. Repetitions: 3 to each side, alternating.

- Breathe deeply and completely.
- Pull with good grip on legs.
- Move slowly—take 4 to 5 seconds for each movement.

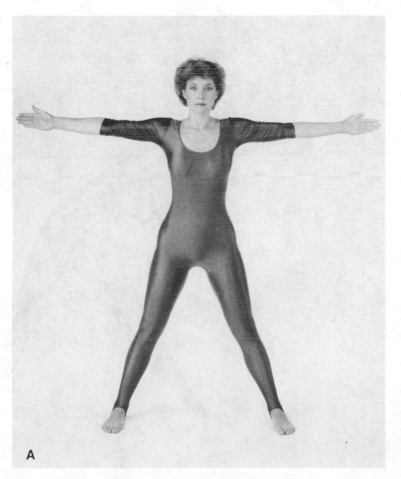

A

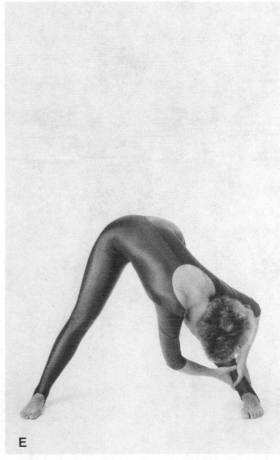

E

SIDE TRIANGLE II, III

(Uttihita Trikonasan)

*Tones muscles of the legs and hips
Stretches and develops the inter-
costal muscles of the rib cage
Helps relieve backaches
Strengthens the neck*

In Courses II and III add this exercise to the warm-up sequence
after the Hip Rock. Stand with
feet apart a comfortable distance,
toes pointed slightly in. Lift arms
straight out to sides (A). Breathe
in and bend to the right, sliding
your right hand down your leg as
far as possible without strain (F).
Grip your leg for support. At the
same time bring your left arm up
and over your head so it is as parallel as possible to the floor and in
a plane with the rest of your body.
Your breath should be all the way
in. Hold for just a moment, then
breathe out and straighten up to
your beginning position, with
arms straight out to the sides.
Repetitions: 3 times on each side.

After you have been practicing
this exercise for at least four
months, you may start holding the
position a little longer. At this
point do not hold your breath in,
but relax and breathe easily in the
position.

- Keep toes pointed in.
- Have upper arm as straight as
  possible parallel to the floor and
  in a plane with the rest of your
  body.

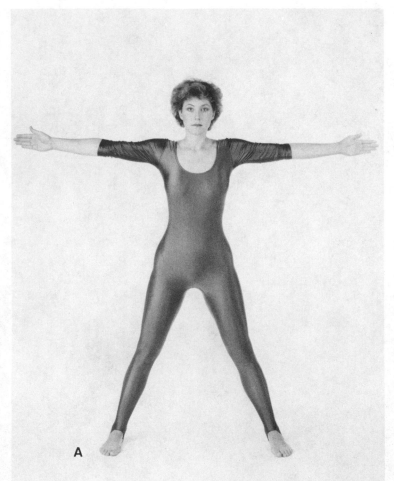

A

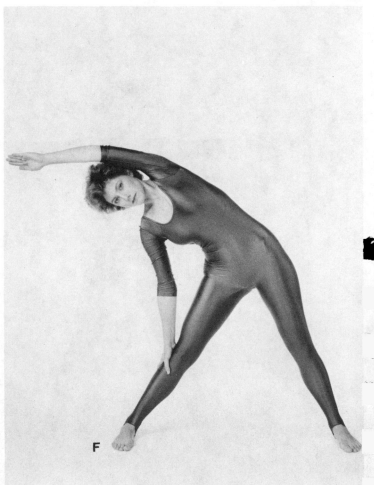

F

TWISTING TRIANGLE II, III
(Parivritta Trikonasan)

Increases flexibility and blood circulation in the lower spine and pelvis
Strengthens hip joints
Invigorates abdominal viscera and diaphragm
Strengthens chest and neck
Helps relieve depression

With legs apart 2 to 3 feet or a comfortable distance, toes pointed in, breathe in and raise arms straight out to the sides (A). Breathe out and bend toward your right leg. Bend from the hip, tilting pelvis forward rather than leading with your head. As you bend, twist your torso downward. Grasp the *outside* of your right calf, ankle or foot with your left hand and pull slightly as you twist even more, raising your right arm straight up (G). Keep your eyes open and look up at your right thumbnail. Hold a second or two and return to a standing position, breathing in as you come up. Move slowly and deliberately.

- Grasp the outside of calf, ankle or foot.
- Breathe out as you twist downward, in as you come up.
- Look at upraised thumbnail.

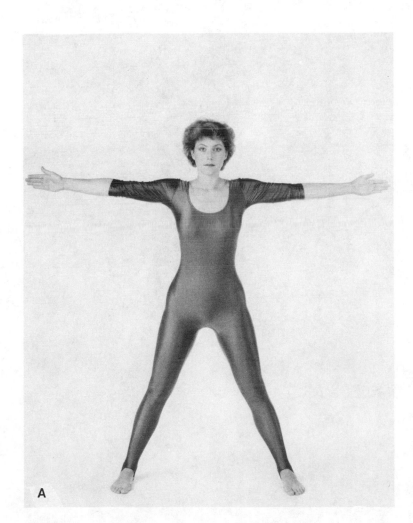

A

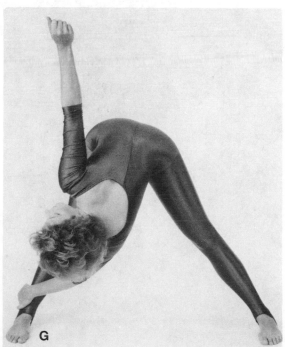

G

WINDMILL II, III

Limbers and strengthens lower spine, hip joints and muscles of upper thigh

Strengthens lungs and breathing muscles and improves respiration

Start with feet apart, toes pointed in, hands supporting lower back with fingers spread (A). Breathe in fully and swivel to the right without moving your feet, so that your torso is facing right (B). Start to breathe out and bend right toward your right leg (C). Bend as far down toward the leg as possible but don't stop; continue moving down and over to your left leg, breathing out (D). At this point your breath should be all the way out. When your head reaches the position of your left leg, start breathing in. Continue breathing in as you straighten up, facing left

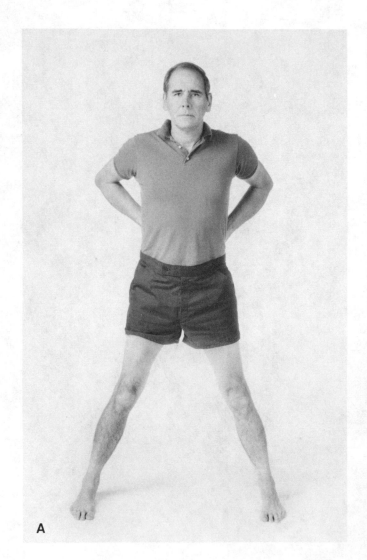

A

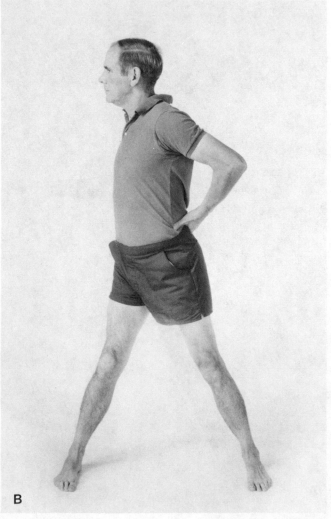

B

(E). When you reach a standing position, your breath should be all the way in and you will be facing left. Hold the breath in as you swivel right and repeat the exercise. Repetitions: 3 times each direction.

Notice that in this exercise your head describes a circle. You breathe out for two-thirds of the circle (from straight up to the second leg) and you breathe in for one-third of the circle (second leg up to straight position). What breath pattern does this remind you of?*

- Breathe in and out completely.
- Swivel completely to each side before and after making the circle.
- Keep knees straight.
- Support lower back with spread fingers.

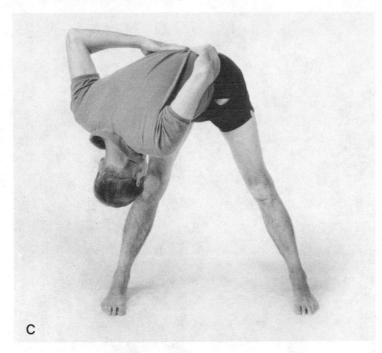

C

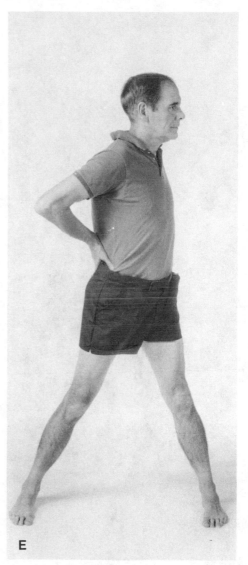

E

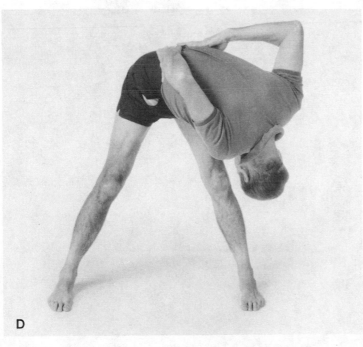

D

*Answer: Humming Breath—short inhalation, long exhalation (p. 138).

TREE POSE I, II
(Vriksasan)

Strengthens legs
Improves concentration and balance
Improves respiration

Stand with feet together. To get the feeling of balancing on one leg, first shift your weight to your left foot and rest your right foot on top of the left. Steady yourself by fixing your gaze on a spot on the wall or floor in front of you. At first hold on to the back of a chair, a bar or the wall—something solid. Now pick up your right foot and place it against the inside of your left leg as high as possible, with the toes pointed toward the floor (A). You may find it easier to hold your foot in place if you are barefoot. If your foot will not go high enough to rest on your inner thigh, just brace it against your knee.

Try to breathe steadily, with *re-*

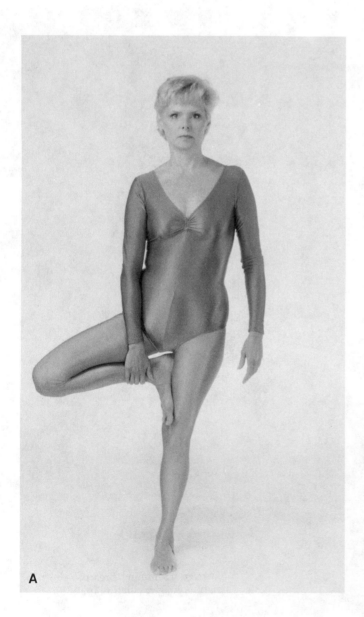

A

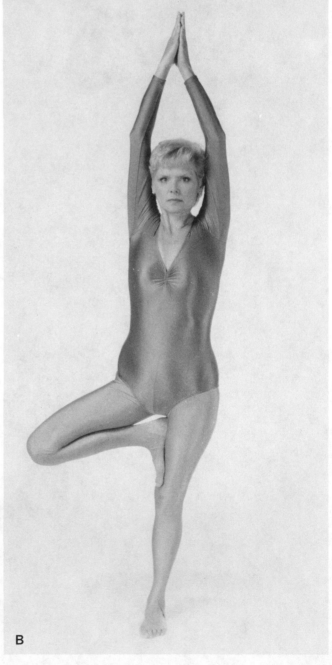

B

laxed stomach muscles the whole time. Because of the extra concentration required to maintain balance, you may find that you will have a tendency to hold your breath. Consciously relax your breath by relaxing your stomach muscles.

When you feel that your balance is steady enough to let go of your chair support, slowly bring your arms straight up overhead with palms together as in the illustration (B). Keep breathing normally. Hold for about 10 seconds at first; work up to 30 seconds or more. Repetitions: 1 each side.

Eventually, as your flexibility increases, your lifted leg will become more parallel to the rest of your body. But in the beginning it's more important to concentrate on maintaining a balanced pose than to worry about the position of the lifted leg. On unsteady days try placing one upraised arm against a wall or door frame to steady yourself.

After you have been practicing for some time, your hips and knees will begin to limber up and you may be able to lift your foot on top of your thigh to do this exercise (C). If so, keep your supporting leg straight and slightly tilt your pelvis forward. As your limberness improves, you will be able to lower your knee toward your supporting leg. Your arms go straight overhead, palms together, as before. This variation strengthens the knee joints.

If you feel very steady, you can try a variation in which you look up slightly as you balance. Be sure to keep your stomach muscles relaxed so that your breath can relax.

- Stare at one spot.
- Relax stomach muscles for relaxed breathing.
- Keep arms straight overhead.

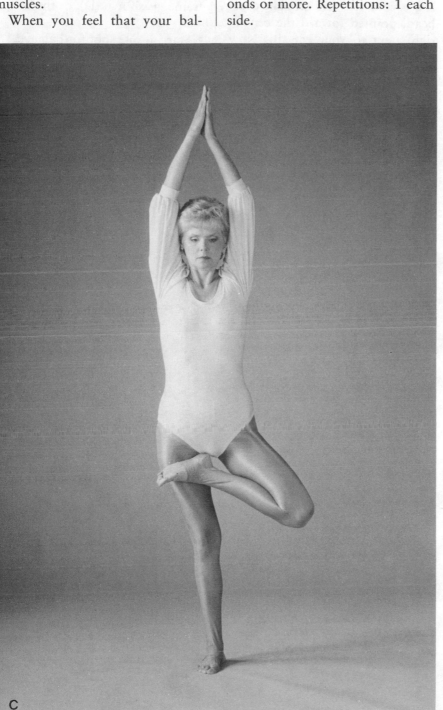

C

DANCER POSE I, II, III

(Natarajasan)

Strengthens lower back and lumbar vertebrae

Stretches and strengthens hips and thighs

Improves balance, poise and concentration

Removes phlegm and opens nasal passages

Improves memory and relieves sluggishness and depression

Those of you with lower back and disk problems should not do this exercise without your doctor's specific approval until your back becomes stronger.

Fix your eyes on one spot for balance. Grasp your left foot firmly with your right hand (A). Raise your left arm straight overhead, pointed toward the ceiling, right next to your ear (B). Now lift your left leg up and back away from your body (not just in toward the buttocks) slowly and carefully (C). Now relax your stomach muscles so that your breath is felt mostly in the diaphragm. Hold the position, relaxing your stomach muscles and breathing easily, for several seconds. Then relax and repeat once on the opposite side. If your balance is shaky, hold on to a door frame, as shown (D), or the wall.

- Stare at one spot for balance.
- Grasp opposite foot.
- Release stomach muscles so that breath relaxes.
- Pull foot up and push it back away from the body.

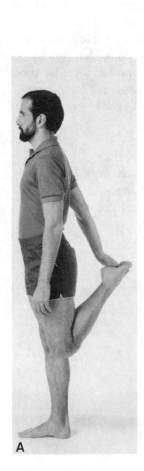

A

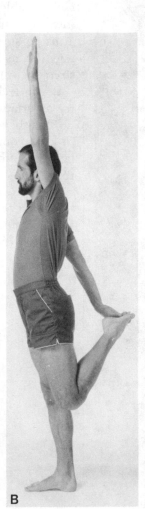

B

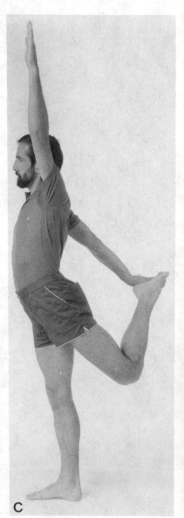

C

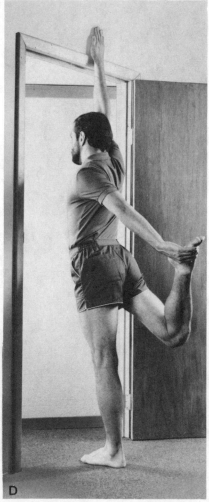

D

T POSE I, II, III
(Virabhadrasan)

Develops very strong legs and back
Improves vigor and agility
Tones abdominal muscles and organs
Increases concentration and mental poise

This exercise is very important for building nervous system strength, improving eyesight and kidney function and reducing anxiety. Holding on to a sturdy chair as in the illustration, step back from the chair about three feet. Lower your torso so that it is parallel to the floor. Raise and lower each leg a few times to warm up and get a feeling for what it feels like to hold your leg parallel to the floor (A).

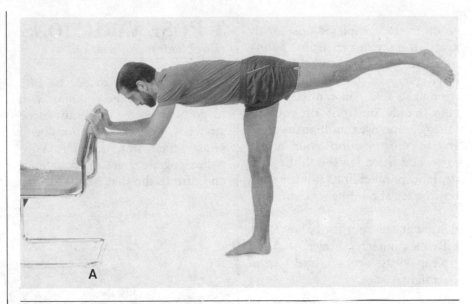

Raise your right leg and bring it as high as you can without bending either of your knees. Now fix your gaze on a spot on the floor, relax your stomach muscles and find your center of balance by gradually releasing your hold on the chair. Bring your palms together with hands pointed straight down toward the floor (B). Hold for a few seconds, then relax and repeat on the other side. Keep your head about half up—not looking straight ahead or straight down.

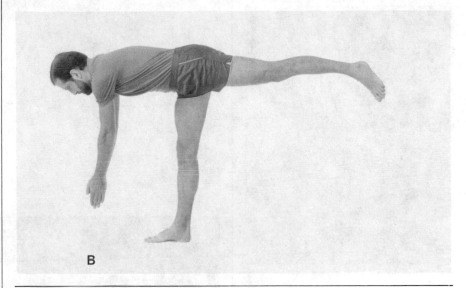

You may also start this exercise by holding on to your right knee with both hands. Stare at one spot, and slowly raise your left leg up in back until it is parallel to the floor or as high as you can lift without straining (C). Keep both knees straight. Then, when you feel steady, release your knees and put your hands together as described before.

After you have practiced this exercise for a few weeks, you can

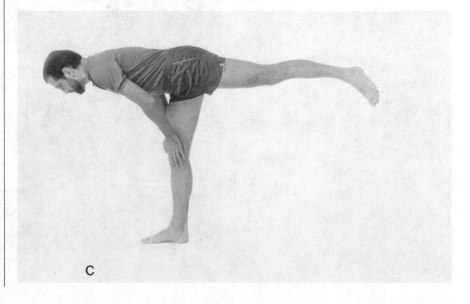

go on to the completed pose, with arms straight out in front, palms together (D). Your head should be lifted very slightly—only high enough so that you can barely see your hands in front of you by raising your eyes as high as they go. In this position your arms, torso and lifted leg should be in a straight, parallel line, and the supporting leg should be straight.

- Stare at one spot for balance.
- Relax stomach muscles.
- Keep legs, torso and arms straight.

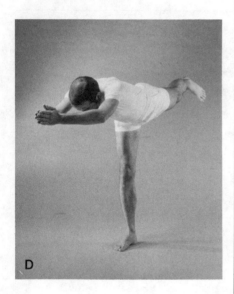

D

T POSE VARIATIONS
(Virabhadrasan Variation)

After practicing these balance poses for some time you may wish to go on to some more advanced stretches. In one variation bend your arms, but, keeping your palms together, get your balance and turn to the side, attempting to bring your arms in a plane with your body (E).

In another variation, the *Stork Stretch* (*Urdhva Prasarita Ekapadasan*), after holding the T Pose, drop your arms so that your fingers, or palms, touch the ground. Your lifted leg stays parallel to the floor (F).

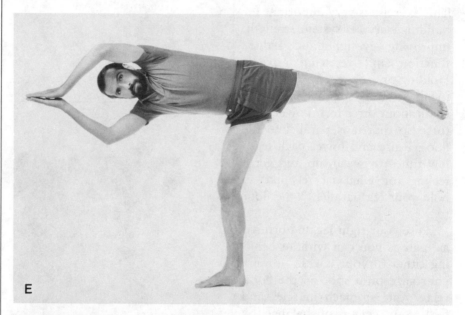

E

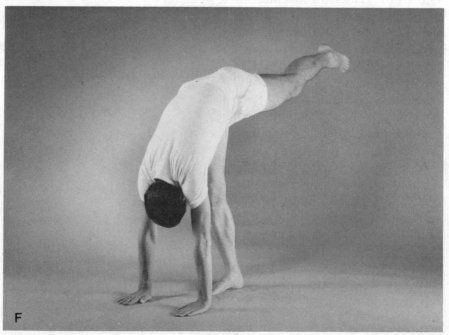

F

T POSE KNEE BENDS II, III

Strengthens hips, knees, lower back and legs
Improves concentration, steadiness and balance

From the T Pose, bring your arms behind your back with fingers clasped (G). Rest them comfortably on your back. Now stare at one spot for balance and gently bend the knee of your supporting leg, just a little. Bend *only a few inches*—this is not meant to be a deep knee bend. Repeat, trying for five repetitions at first. After several weeks you may increase to ten repetitions. If balance is a little unsteady, use a chair for support (H).

• Keep hands loosely clasped behind back.
• Keep breathing relaxed.

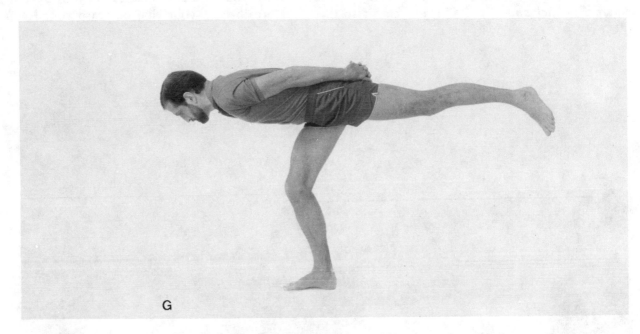

G

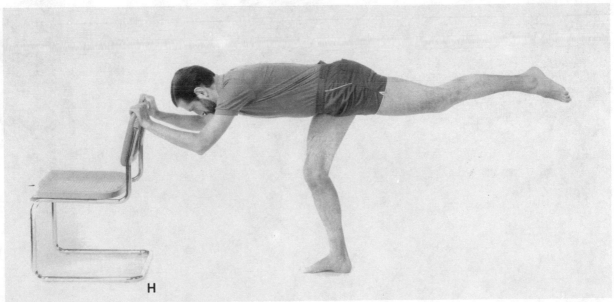

H

STANDING SUN POSE I, II, III

(Padahasthasan)

Stimulates and improves all activities of the stomach, liver, spleen and abdominal region
Improves circulation
Strengthens and relieves tension and stress on heart and lungs
Limbers and strengthens muscles and nerves of back and legs

Stand straight, feet parallel, and breathe out (A). Breathe in as you raise your arms to the sides in a semicircle (B) and then overhead. Stretch and look up (C). Then start to breathe out and bend forward from the hips, keeping your head between your arms (D). Try to match your breath to your movement so that your breath is not all the way out until you are all the way down. Holding your breath out, grasp your legs firmly with both hands; bend your elbows, keeping your arms close to your sides, and pull your upper body gently toward your legs (E). Remember not to use stomach or back muscles. If you can't bend your elbows, grasp your legs far-

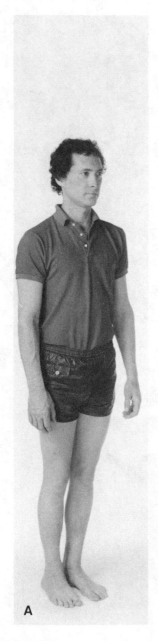

A

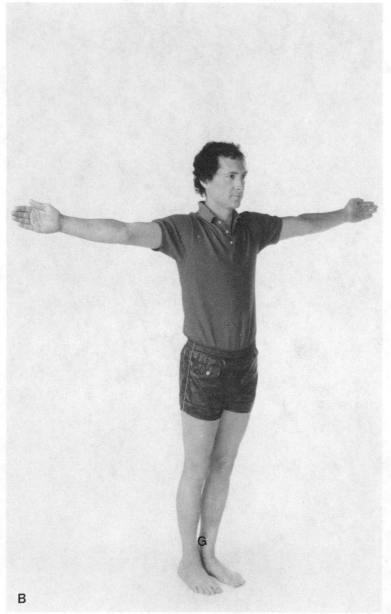

B

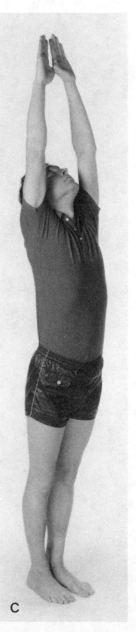

C

ther up until you can bend them. Now release your legs and begin to breathe in and straighten up, keeping your arms loose at first and then out to the sides (F) and overhead again, so that your breath is all the way in when your arms are overhead. Then breathe out and lower your arms to your sides. Relax. Repetitions: 3.

When you are more limber, you may be able to pull your upper body even farther toward your legs (G).

Unlike the other forward-bending poses learned so far, this exercise does not have the continuous up-and-down pumping motion. Instead you must lower the arms between each repetition.

- Keep knees straight.
- Pull by bending elbows, not by tensing stomach or back.
- Coordinate movement with breath.
- Bend slowly.

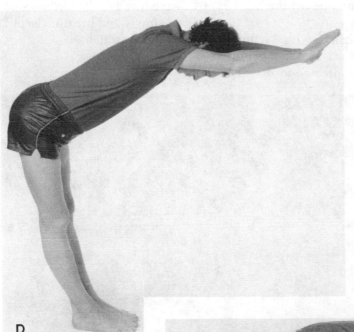

D

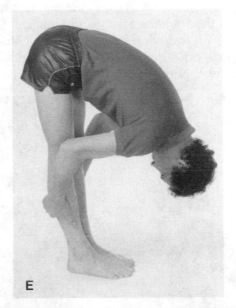

E

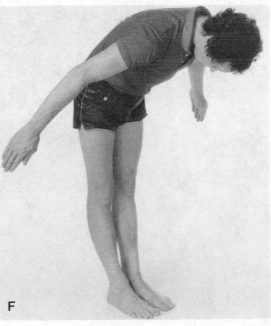

F

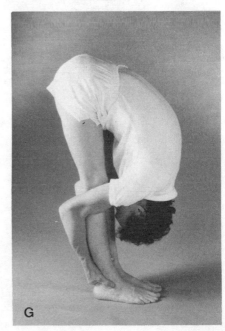

G

SUN POSE VARIATION III
(Parsvottanasan)

*Lubricates and limbers shoulder
  joints and shoulder blades, lum-
  bar vertebrae and neck*
*Gives an intense stretch to entire
  chest, lungs and heart*
Corrects breathing difficulties
Tones abdominal organs
Strengthens legs and back
Improves posture

This variation of the Standing Sun Pose is for those of you who are rather limber and can attempt a more challenging pose. Your hands are clasped and interlocked behind your back, palms together, and your arms are straightened and flexed up and away from the body. This position of flexing the arms behind the back is common to several other advanced yoga asans. It limbers the entire upper back muscles and joints, as well as stretching the rib cage and lungs, allowing more fresh blood into the nerves and tissues of the heart and lungs.

Stand straight, with hands clasped and arms locked behind your back (H). Breathe in deeply, then exhale slowly, bending at the hips. As you bend, flex the arms up and away from your back. Bend forward as far as possible, bringing your upper body close to your legs without bending your knees (I). Hold this position with the breath out for a second or two, then breathe in slowly and come up. Repetitions: 3.

- Clasp hands and lock elbows.
- Bend slowly and breathe deeply.
- Keep knees straight.

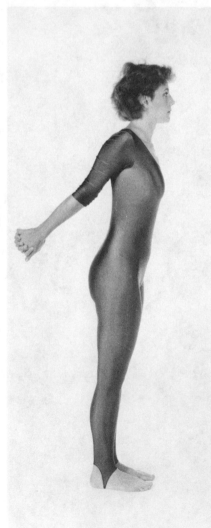

H

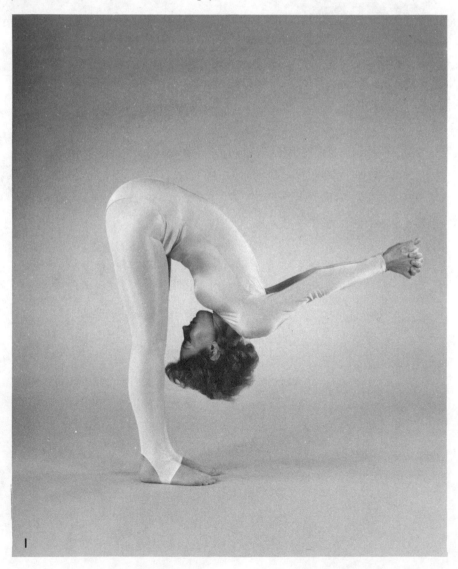

I

ARM AND LEG BALANCE I, II, III

Strengthens hip joints
Improves balance
Promotes correct posture
Strengthens shoulders and upper back

Starting from hands and knees, breathe in and slowly raise your right arm and left leg (A). Try to lift the arm straight out in front and the leg straight out in back, both parallel to the floor. Hold for a second, looking at the tip of your middle finger, then breathe out and lower. Repeat with left arm and right leg. If your balance is a bit shaky at first, look down and pick a spot on the floor for balance. Repetitions: 3 on each side, alternating sides.

In a variation of this exercise, raise the right arm and right leg (B), trying not to lean to the side, but keeping the back as straight and level as possible. Repetitions: 3 on each side, alternating sides.

- Breathe slowly and deeply, coordinating breath with movement.
- Gaze at a spot on the floor for balance, or at the tip of your outstretched middle finger.

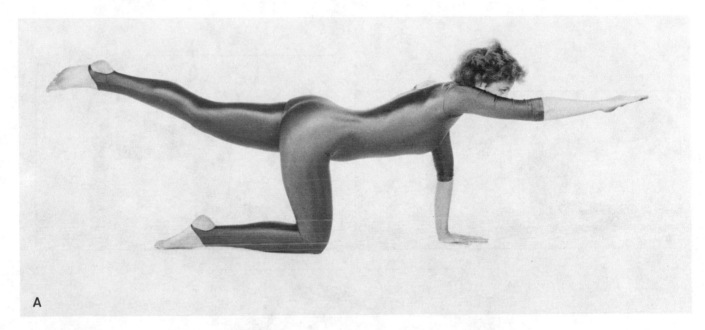

A

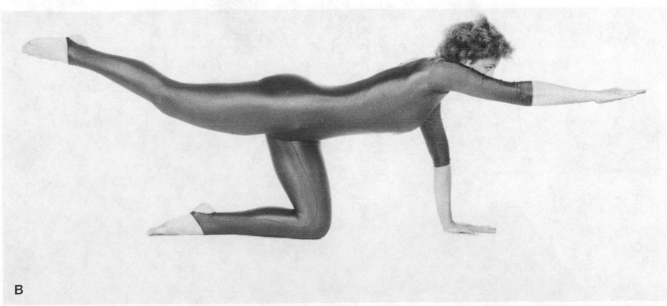

B

CAT BREATH I, II, III

Improves the action of intestines, heart, lungs and liver

Purifies blood

Helps in management of hypertension

Limbers spinal column and relieves tension in lower back

Improves respiration and breathing muscles

Start on hands and knees (A). Breathe in slowly and deeply, arching your back and looking up (B). Then breathe out deeply and tuck your head, rounding your back so your spine bends in the opposite direction (C). Repetitions: 3 to 5.

- Breathe deeply and smoothly.
- Coordinate breath with movement of spine.

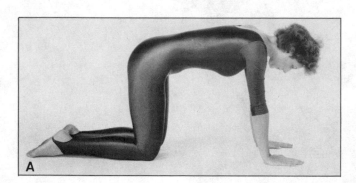

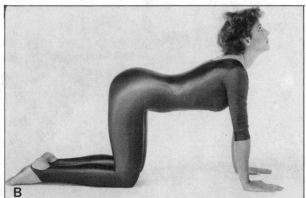

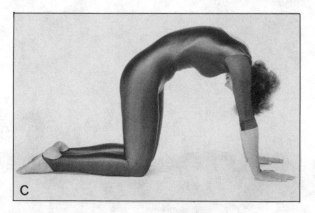

CAT BREATH VARIATION III

Breaks up tensed breathing patterns
Strengthens upper back, shoulder and hip joints
Limbers lower spine

This exercise is part of the Emotional Stability Routine (Course Three). It involves using a "double breath," meaning that the breath is manipulated by the natural movement of the body. Start on hands and knees and breathe in (A). Breathe out as you tuck your head and bring your right knee up toward your forehead (D). This is a natural breath because of the compression on your midsection when you bring your forehead and knee close together. Now breathe in as you raise your head and bring your leg back (E). Continue lifting your leg in back as high as possible, while breathing out and simultaneously bending your elbows and arching your back so that your chin comes toward the floor (F). This is a compression in the opposite direction and also is a natural out-breath. As you gain proficiency in this breath pattern, you can speed up the movement. Repetitions: 3 to 6 with each leg.

- Breathe *out* in the extreme up and extreme down positions, and breathe *in* during the transitions in between.

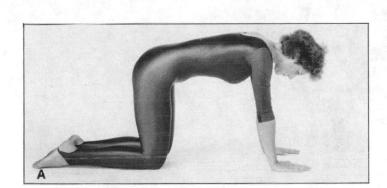

A

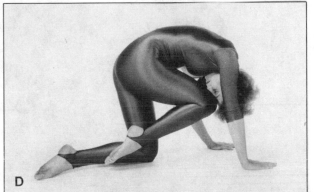

D

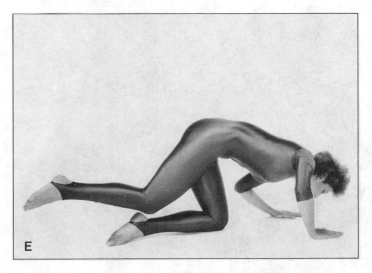

E

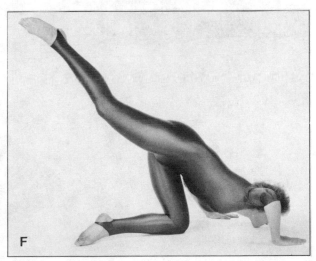

F

BOW VARIATION I, II

(Dhanurasan Var.)

*Strengthens vertebrae, back muscles, hips, thighs and shoulders
Improves balance and memory*

Starting on hands and knees, reach back and grasp your *left* foot with your *right* hand (G). Lift the leg as high as you can, arching your back if possible. Hold for several seconds, breathing normally. Repetitions: 1 on each side.

Then, reach back and grasp the *right* foot with the *right* hand (H). Repeat once on the other side.

- Keep balance by staring at one spot on the floor.
- Lift the foot as high as possible.
- Keep breath relaxed; don't hold your breath.

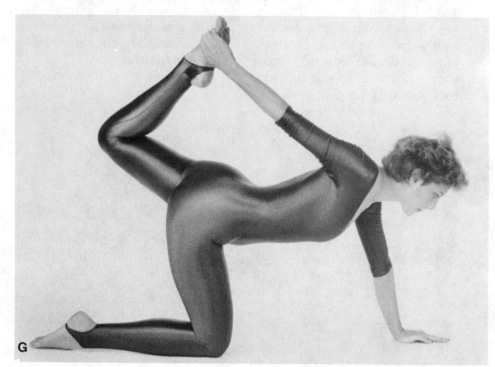

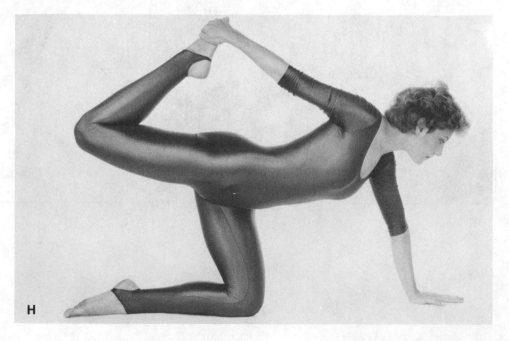

COBRA V-RAISE II, III

Strengthens legs, upper back, shoulders and intercostal muscles of the rib cage

Limbers and strengthens chest, neck, abdomen and groin

Improves functioning of the organs in the pelvic region through increased blood flow, improving reproductive function

Reduces body fat

This is a combination pose for Course Two requiring extra strength and stamina. In this exercise only the hands and feet touch the floor. It can be started from a standing position, by leaning forward and "walking" the hands out in front into position, or from a hands-and-knees position. Begin by exhaling and pushing the buttocks into the air, tucking your head and pushing your heels down toward the floor so that your body looks like an inverted V (A). Then breathe in as you lower your hips and arch your back, looking up (B). Try to keep your legs straight, knees not touching the floor, if possible. Repetitions: 3 to 6.

For an even greater challenge try this exercise on your fingertips. This strengthens the wrists, forearms and hands in addition to the already-mentioned benefits.

- Breathe deeply, and coordinate breath with movement.
- Remember to tuck head on exhalation.

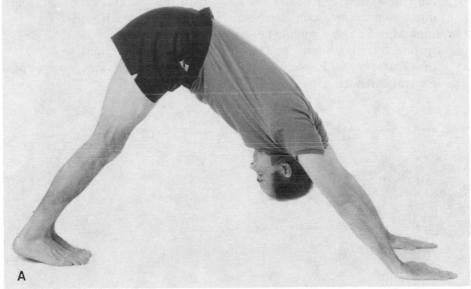

A

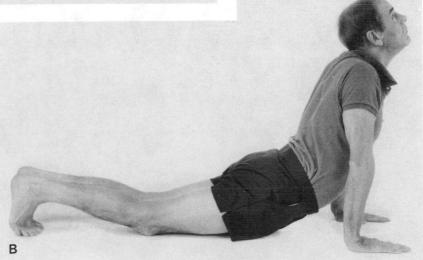

B

FORWARD AND SIDE PLANK III

Strengthens wrists, arms, shoulders and neck
Improves circulation to entire upper body
Strengthens back muscles

This is another demanding series for Course Three. In this exercise most of the body's muscles are being used, and it will be very tempting to want to hold your breath. However, you must try to let your breath go into its own natural pattern, the Easy Breath pattern, which will be shorter and more forceful—rather like panting. Even though you are using most of your body's strength in this exercise, you should still try to relax your stomach muscles so that your *body* decides how to breathe. Because of the extra demand on the body, you'll find that your breath naturally becomes faster and heavier, in order for more oxygen to reach the muscles.

From the V-raise, or from hands and knees, straighten the legs and position your hips so that your legs and torso make a straight line. Lean on your left hand and lift your right arm out in front of you, extending the line (A). At first you may not be strong enough to support your whole body's weight on one hand. If so, just practice *leaning* on one hand at a time, back and forth, until your arms gain strength. Look ahead at your middle fingertip and let your breath go. Hold for a few seconds. Repeat with the left arm extended.

Next, lean on your left arm again and raise your right arm up overhead, turning your head to look at your thumbnail (B). Your body will be twisted sideways, including both feet. Hold for a few seconds, letting your breath go. Relax and repeat with the left arm extended.

After practicing these variations separately for a few weeks, you may do them in sequence. Start with the Forward Plank, raising your right arm forward, then immediately bring the arm up overhead for the Side Plank. Repeat with the left arm extended. Repetitions: 1 on each side.

• Keep body straight.
• Let breath relax as much as possible.

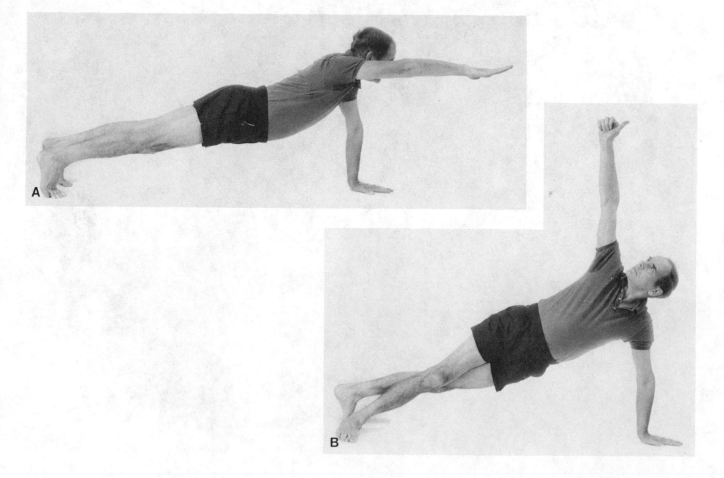

HERO POSE VARIATION II
(Virasan Variation)

Helps strengthen arches of people with flat feet

Relieves stiffness in hips, knees and ankles

Relieves bloatedness in stomach and intestines

Improves breathing and circulation in entire pelvic region, especially toning kidneys and reproductive organs; may improve reproductive function

Improves flexibility in lower back and hips

Reduces body fat from sides and thighs

Sit on your feet with your arms overhead, one hand on top of the other (A). Breathe in deeply while rising off your feet a few inches, then begin to exhale and slide to the left (B). Finish exhaling as you sit down. Try to keep your knees on the floor as you move. Now breathe in and lift up again and over to the right, exhaling as you sit down. If your legs are not strong enough to do this exercise at first, support yourself minimally with one hand on either side, trying to use your leg muscles as much as possible. Repetitions: 3 to each side, finishing by coming back to the center.

- Try to keep back straight and knees on the floor.
- Breathe in as you come up, breathe out as you sit down.

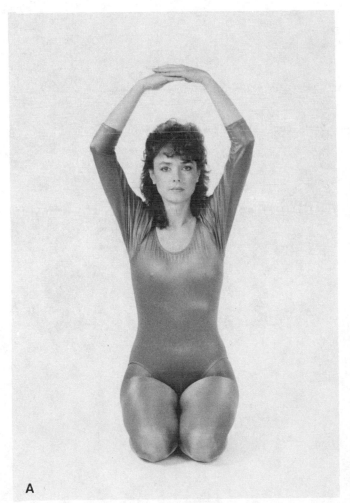

A

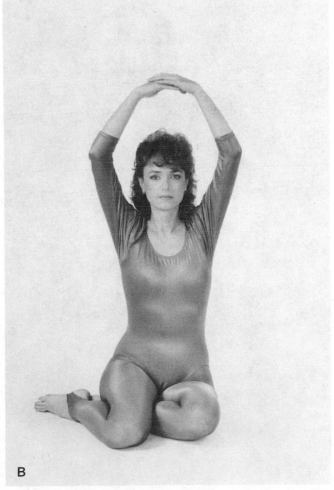

B

EXTENDED HERO POSE II

(Virasan Extension)

Increases circulation to head
Oxygenates and purifies blood
Strengthens shoulders, ankles and
*　chest and improves posture*
Limbers intercostal muscles

Clasp your hands and fingers behind your back and lock your elbows, straightening your arms (C). Your toes should be just touching and your ankles spread apart so as to form a seat for the buttocks. Breathe in deeply, then exhale completely as you bend forward. Raise the arms up and away from the body (D); hold this position for a second, then breathe in, come back up to a seated position and relax. Repetitions: 3.

- Keep hands clasped and arms straight.
- Breathe in and out deeply.

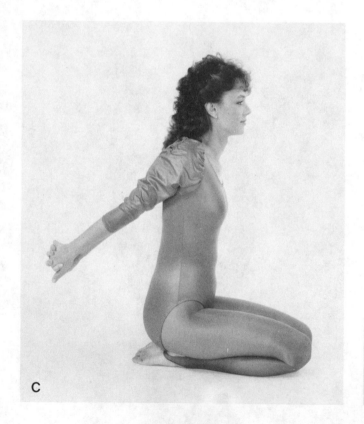

C

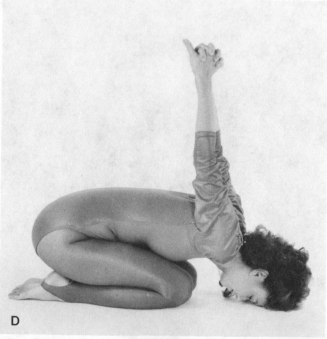

D

ANKLE STRETCH II

Limbers and strengthens ankles, hips and knees
Strengthens abdominal muscles

Sit on your feet, arms at your sides, breathing normally (A).

Gently lift your knees up as far as possible, while pushing down slightly with your fingers if necessary to intensify the lift (B). Lower your knees and relax. Repetitions: 3.

- Breathe normally—don't hold your breath.
- Lift knees high enough to stretch ankles, but do not strain.

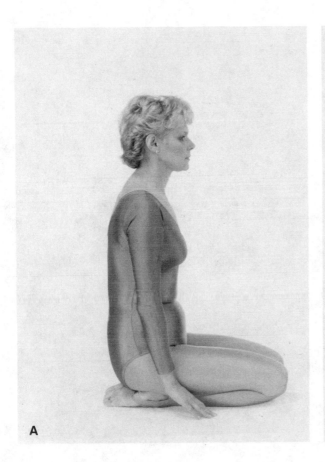

A

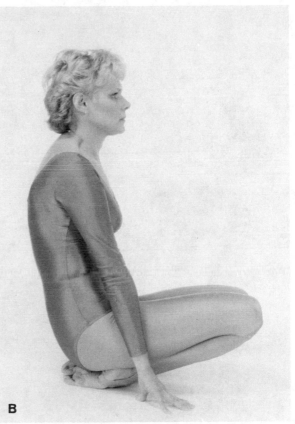

B

CAMEL POSE II

Limbers entire spine and pelvis; opens chest, improving respiration

Improves circulation in spinal column

Stretches and strengthens upper and lower thigh and knees

For this Course Two exercise start in a kneeling position. The first illustration shows a warm-up to this intense stretch. Lean back with your right hand and grasp your right heel with your right hand (A). Push your hips forward until you feel the muscles being stretched across the pelvis and thighs. Now release, relax and repeat on the other side. Finally, lean back and grasp both heels. Gently tilt your head back, being careful not to strain your neck, and keeping your teeth together, push your hips forward, as if someone had a rope around your waist and was pulling forward (B). Hold the position for a few seconds, breathing normally. You should notice your breath moving mostly in the belly area, using the breath pattern called the Easy Breath (see p. fill). Repetitions: 1 on each side for the warm-up, and just once for the completed pose.

- Keep teeth together.
- Push hips forward, stretching thighs and strengthening knees.
- Breathe gently from the belly.

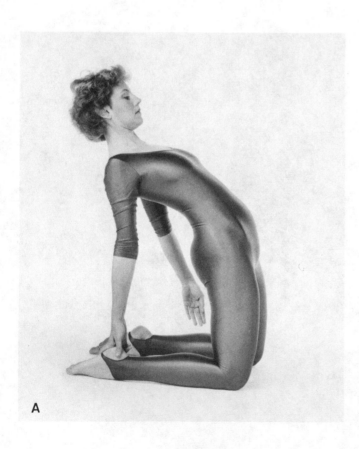

A

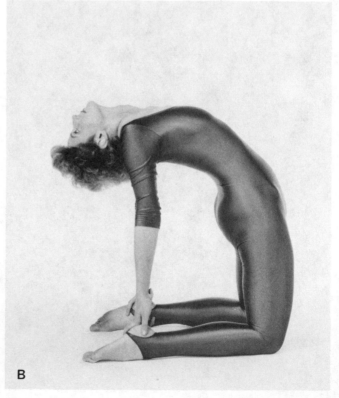

B

THIGH STRETCH II, III
(Hanumanasan Preparation)

Stretches and strengthens abductor muscles of thighs and hips
Increases blood circulation to pelvis
Improves reproductive function
Elongates nerves and muscles in the legs

This is an effective exercise for runners because it stretches the hamstrings and groin muscles. Start by kneeling on your right knee with your toes flat. Your right thigh should be at a 45-degree angle to the floor. Bend your left knee, foot flat on the floor and calf perpendicular to the floor. Your fingertips rest on the floor beside your left foot (A). Breathe in and lean forward, arching your back and looking up (B). Then breathe out and sit back, straightening your left leg and bending your head forward toward your left knee (C). Keep the toes of your left foot pointed straight ahead. Repetitions: 3 each side.

- Breathe deeply and smoothly, matching breath with movement.
- Do not strain beyond your limits.

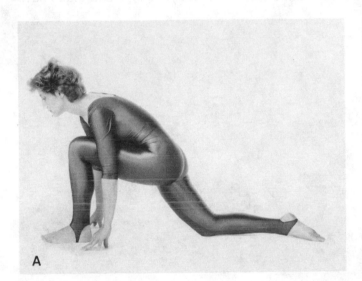

A

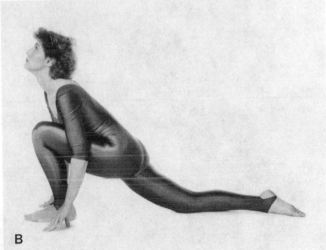

B

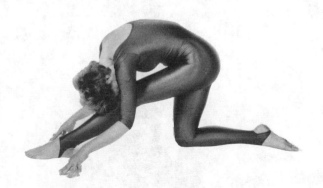

C

PIGEON POSE II, III

(Rajakapotasan)

Stretches, strengthens and tones spinal column and all spinal muscles and nerves, especially cervical and sacral vertebrae

Strengthens and limbers hip joints and groin muscles

Stimulates metabolic and reproductive glands and organs

Increases vitality

May relieve impotence

Strengthens and stretches rib cage and chest

Start by sitting on your heels (A). Slide your right leg back, keeping the top of your knee on the floor so that your hip and leg do not twist to the side. You should be sitting directly on top of your left foot. Place your palms next to your left knee and rest your chest on your thigh, forehead to the floor (B). Breathe out completely. Start breathing in and curl your head back as far as possible, keeping your eyes looking straight up through your forehead. Continue breathing in and raise your chest, keeping the spine curled, and then the stomach. Come up on your fingertips to give yourself a further arch to the spine (C). Hold for a second or two, then start to breathe out and lower your body in reverse order: stomach first, then chest, keeping your head back; then finally lower your head after your chest is resting again on your thigh. Repetitions: 3 each side.

After your hips and knees have

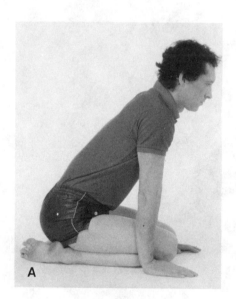

A

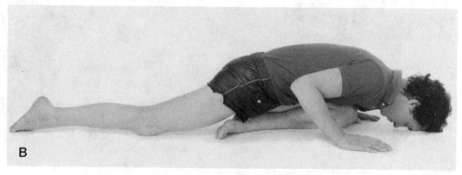

B

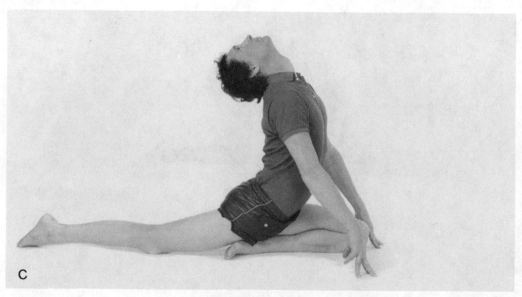

C

become more limber, you may try this exercise with your front leg turned out to the side, so that your front foot is resting on its side (D). The back leg must still be placed so that the top of the knee is on the floor.

When the curriculum instructs you to hold the Pigeon Pose, push up on your fists after your third repetition and tuck your toes under in back (E). Fix your gaze to a spot on the floor about three feet to the front (do *not* look up in this hold—your neck must remain straight). Relax your stomach muscles, breathe normally and hold the pose for 10 to 30 seconds.

A further variation is shown in which you begin in the starting position with your fingers clasped behind your back and arms locked. Use the same breath pattern. In this variation much more back strength is required (F). You can try for even a further stretch by bending your knee in back and bringing your pointed toes as close to your head as possible as you arch up (G).

- Look up and keep teeth together.
- Curl and uncurl your spine.
- Use your hands for support but not as a push-up.

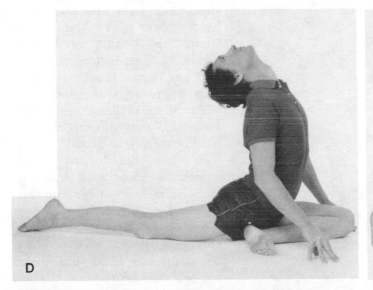

D

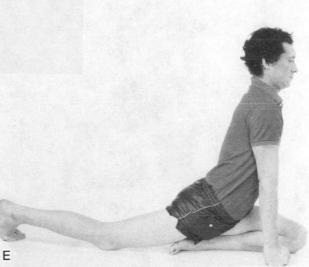

E

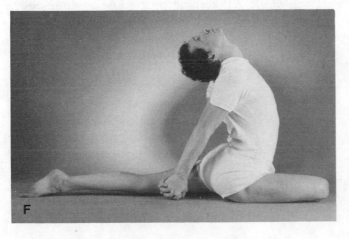

F

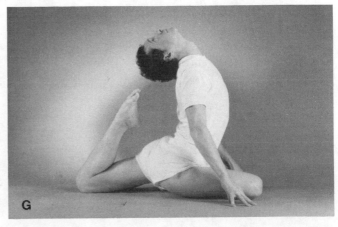

G

FOOT FLAPS I

Limbers ankles and toes
Improve mind-body coordination
Gently warms up sciatic nerve and muscles in back of legs in preparation for forward-bending poses
May relieve bedsores and varicose veins
Reduces body fat in thighs and hips

Sit with legs straight in front of you. Make fists and pull your toes back toward your face as far as you can without strain (A). Now open your hands and push your feet forward, away from your face (B). Repeat several times. Now open your right hand and make a fist with your left, while pushing right toes forward and pulling left toes back. Alternate and repeat several times. Then grab hold of your legs and rotate your ankles in circles: both one way, then the other, then opposite ways.

- Keep knees straight.
- Breathe normally.

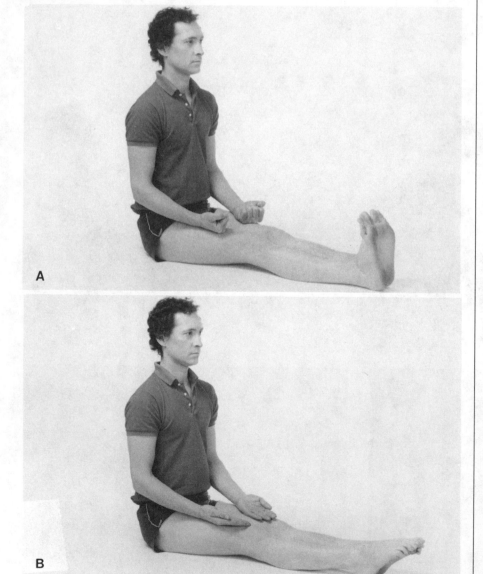

SEATED SUN POSE
I, II
(Paschimottanasan)

Strengthens abdominal viscera and diaphragm
Improves digestive function; helps relieve constipation
Excellent for diabetics
Tones sympathetic nervous system and nerves in back of legs
Strengthens and stretches legs and spine
May help relieve impotence

Start with both legs out in front of you, feet flexed back toward your face, back straight and arms at your sides (A). Breathe out completely. Now start to breathe in and bring your arms in a wide circle to the sides and over your head. Lock your thumbs and stretch up, looking up at your hands (B). This will open the rib cage and improve breathing. Now start to breathe out and bend from the hips, tilting your pelvis forward slightly and keeping your head between your arms (C). Keep your feet flexed and knees straight. Bend forward from the waist as far as you can comfortably and grasp your legs firmly at the knees, calves or ankles. By now you should have breathed out completely. Hold your breath out as you bend your elbows, keeping them close to your body, and gently pull your upper body down toward your legs (D). Do not bounce or strain. If you can't bend your elbows, grab your legs up farther toward your knees or thighs until you can. Hold this position with the breath out for a second or two, then breathe in and relax your arms, letting them be pulled back as you start to straighten, then bring your arms to the sides and up in a wide circle again as before, breathing in all the way to the top. Lock your thumbs, stretch up and look up at your hands. Then breathe out and lower your arms slowly to your sides and relax. If you have a weak back, you can do this exercise seated with your back against the wall.

If you can reach your toes and still bend your elbows easily, you are already quite limber in your hips and the back of your legs! Grab your toes so that your thumb and forefinger on each hand are touching your big toe, as shown (E). (The completed pose is shown in the final photo F.) This completes a nerve circuit in your body and will enhance the effectiveness of the exercise.

- Keep knees straight, feet flexed.
- Breathe in and out completely, coordinating the breath with the movement.
- Do not bounce.
- Be sure breath is all the way out at the bottom hold.
- Bend from hips, not waist.

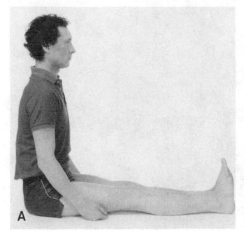

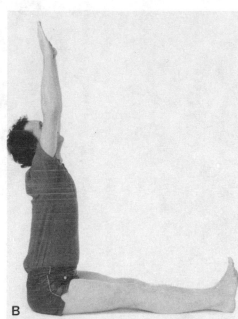

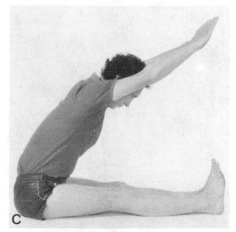

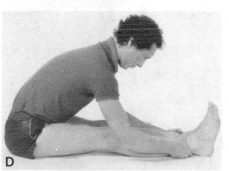

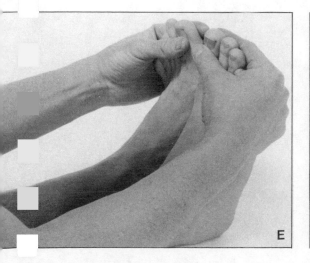

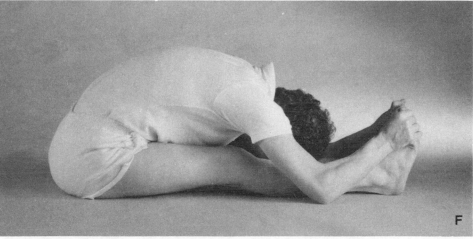

SUN POSE BALANCE
II
(Paschimottanasan Variation)

Strengthens abdominal muscles
Increases circulation in pelvis
Strengthens hip joints and legs
Develops mental stability

The most important objective in this exercise is to retain balance.

Start by grabbing your ankles or toes with your hands (A). Then lean back a little and find your center of balance. Slowly try to straighten your legs (B) and pull your head as far forward as possible (C). Hold the position for several seconds, breathing normally. You may have to support yourself with a folded blanket or towel under your buttocks.

• Find your balance before straightening your legs.
• Don't hold your breath.

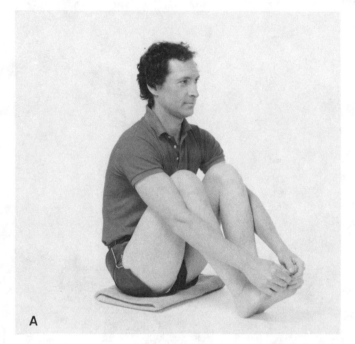

A

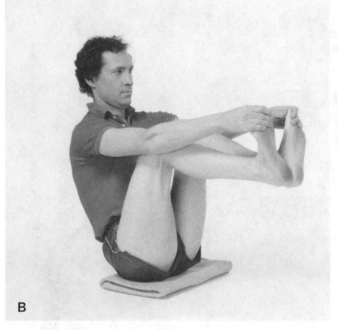

B

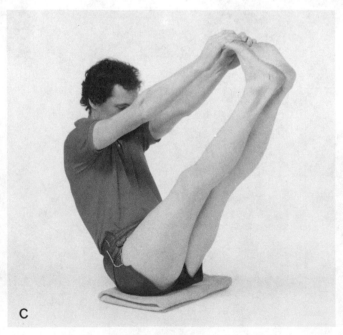

C

ALTERNATE SEATED SUN POSE I, II, III
(Paschimottanasan)

Same benefits as for the Seated Sun Pose

Start with both legs straight out in front. Bend your right knee and massage the knee for several seconds to warm and relax the joint (A). Supporting the knee with your hand, gently lower it to the floor, and with your other hand place the sole of your right foot against your left inner thigh as high as possible (B). Flex the toes of your outstretched leg back toward your face. Sit up straight, arms at your sides, and exhale completely. Breathe in, bringing your arms in a wide circle to the sides and overhead. Lock your thumbs and stretch up, looking up at your hands (C). Start to breathe out as you bend forward from the hips, keeping your head between your arms. Bend forward as far as you can without strain. Grab the outstretched leg with both hands, bend your elbows and pull your upper body toward your leg (D). Your breath should be completely out. Hold for a second or two, then start to breathe in, letting your arms relax and be pulled back; then bring your arms in another wide circle overhead. Lock your thumbs, stretch and look up, then relax and breathe out, bringing your arms back down to the sides. Repetitions: 3 times to each side.

Just as in the Seated Sun Pose, if you can reach your toes and still bend your elbows, grab your big toe with both hands.

After your hip joint becomes more limber, you may try this exercise with your foot on top of your thigh (E); however, if your knee is more than 3 or 4 inches off the floor, you should wait and instead practice the Limber Hips exercise (following) often. If you put your foot on top of your thigh, be sure that the whole foot, not just the toes, is resting on the thigh.

- Bend from the hips, not the waist.
- Breathe slowly and completely, matching breath with movement.
- Keep toes flexed on outstretched leg.

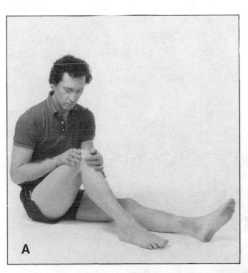

A

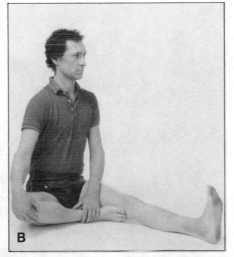

B

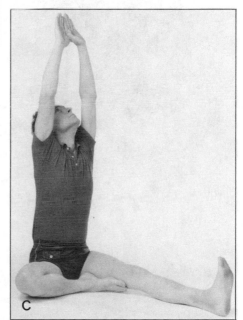

C

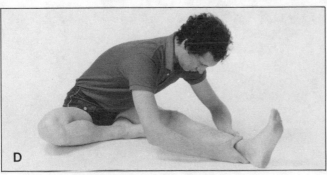

D

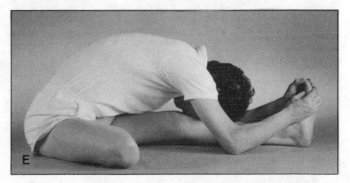

E

LIMBER HIPS I

Limbers hip and knee joints

This exercise helps prepare you for a more comfortable seated position. After the Alternate Sun Pose, support your bent knee, pick up your foot and place the foot on top of the outstretched leg (A). Lean back on your opposite hand (if right foot is on left leg, lean back on left hand). With the other hand gently press down on the bent knee and release several times. Do not press to the point of pain! This is an exercise you can do at various times of the day to work on loosening the knee and hip joints.

When your hips and knees have become more limber, pick up the knee and foot as illustrated and pull the foot close to your chest (B). Then move the foot over to one ear (as if it were a telephone!) and then the other.

- Breathe normally.
- Press down and pull up gently on the bent knee.

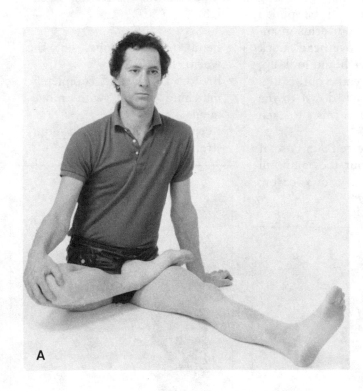

A

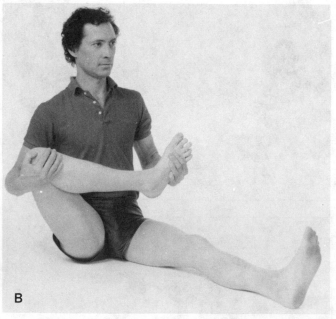

B

EASY SPINE TWIST
I

Gently limbers spine in preparation for full Spine Twist
Improves digestion and eyesight
Tones nerves of spine

Sit cross-legged, tailor fashion. Place your left hand on the floor behind your left hip, straightening your left arm, and place your right hand on the outside of your left knee. Straighten your back and look forward. Breathe in completely. Then breathe out and twist toward the left, keeping your head straight, following a horizontal line at eye level around the room as far left as you can (A). Hold the position for several sec-onds, breathing gently, then release and come back around to the front. Repeat to the right.

In a variation of this exercise, straighten your right leg and bend your left leg, lifting the left foot over on the opposite side of your right leg near the knee. With your right hand, reach through the lifted knee and grasp your thigh on the outside. You'll be able to pull with this hand to twist far-ther. Place your left hand on the floor behind your left hip. Straighten your back (straightening your left arm will help) and look forward, breathing in. Breathe out as you twist left as far as possible, fixing your gaze on a spot at eye level on the wall (B). Hold for several seconds, breathing gently, then release. Repeat on opposite side.

In any lateral twist to the spine, it is important to keep your back and head erect. If you slouch or bend your head before twisting, you will end up with a spiral instead of a side twist.

- Keep spine and head erect.
- Breathe normally when holding the pose.
- Exert a little pull with the forward hand to increase the twist.

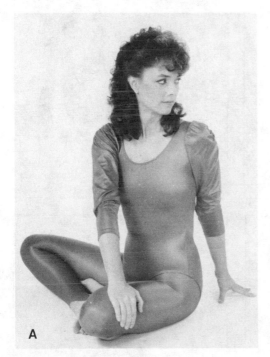

A

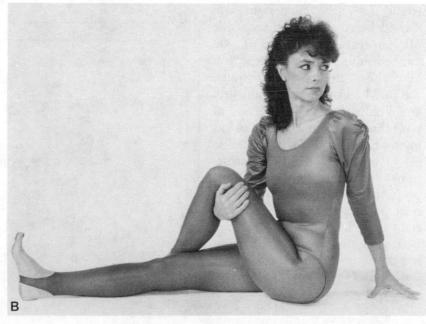

B

SPINE TWIST I, II, III

(Ardha Matsyendrasan)

Relieves chronic constipation
Helps relieve urinary, bladder and
*   prostate difficulties*
Strengthens rib cage and chest
Improves digestion
Tones spinal nerves from base of
*   spine to eyes*
Limbers hips and shoulders

Start with both legs bent at the knee in front (A). Weave your right leg through the left, so the right knee rests on the floor and the right foot is curled beside the left hip (B). Place your left foot on the outside of your right knee (C). You will always be twisting to the opposite side of the raised leg. Before twisting, always make sure that your spine is straight with the following check: Lean back on both hands and arch your spine slightly, keeping your head forward so as not to strain your neck (D). Now straighten your spine up and twist to the left, lifting your rib cage and placing both hands on the floor beside your back (right) foot (E). Your right arm should be entirely on the outside of your raised (left) leg. If you have trouble with this step, you may substitute reaching through the lifted leg with your right arm and holding on to the outside of your thigh with your right hand as in the Easy Spine Twist variation (F). Continue with the instructions that follow, starting with the position of the left hand in the next paragraph.) Now bend your right arm, lift your rib cage and, with your elbow, gently push your left knee back and forth a few times (G). Now push it back as far as it will go, straighten your arm and grasp your pant leg, your

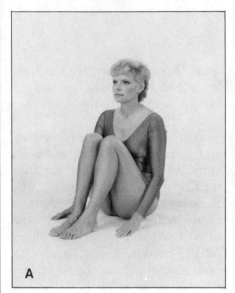

A

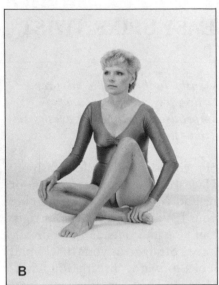

B

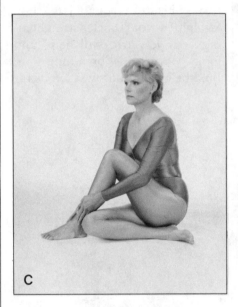

C

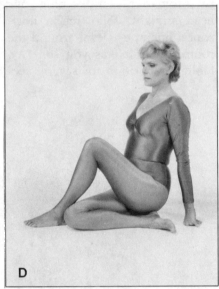

D

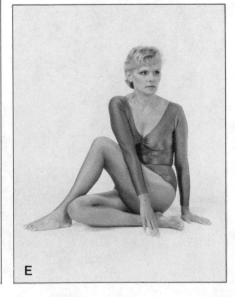

E

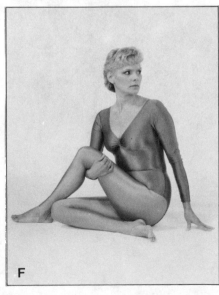

F

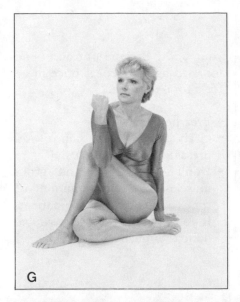

G

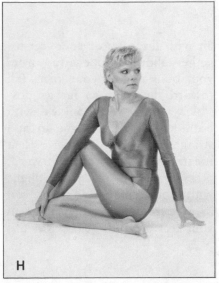

H

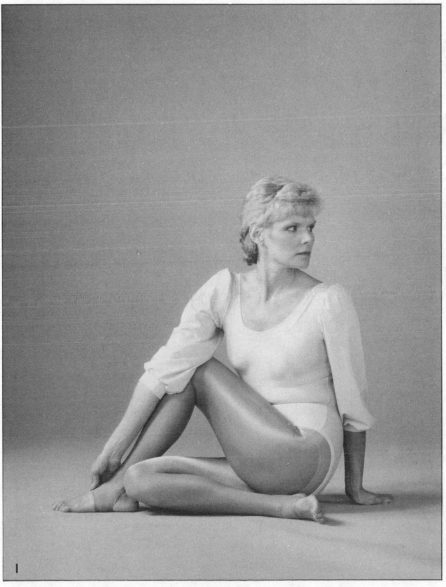

I

right knee (H), or your left ankle, if you are very limber. The important thing is to keep that right arm on the outside of your left knee. That arm is a lever that twists the right side of your body as far to the left as possible.

Now place your left hand behind you at the base of your spine, straightening your arm. If you wish, bend the arm and be on your fingertips. You may point your fingers in toward your body or away from yourself slightly, but the important thing to remember about the position of this back support hand is that it should be *as close to the end of your spine as possible.* This is because your back—all the way from the base of your spine to your neck—must be perfectly straight so that it receives a real lateral stretch. If your hand is too far away from you, your back will curve into a slouch and your spine will be bent in a sort of spiral shape. The lower back area is especially likely to slouch, so before you twist, pull yourself up out of your rib cage and straighten your lower back by pushing your pelvis slightly forward and straightening your support arm. Straighten your spine, look forward and breathe in. Breathe out and twist to the left, keeping your head erect and eyes focused on a spot at eye level as far to the left as you can see comfortably (I). Hold the position for several seconds, breathing gently. Then release, and switch sides. Repetitions: 1 each side.

- Keep spine and head erect.
- Breathe normally.
- Focus eyes on one spot.

DIAMOND POSE
WARM-UP I, II
(Bhadrasan)

Strengthens and limbers hip joints
Relieves urinary difficulties
Helps prevent susceptibility to hernia
Helps relieve prostate difficulties
Tones entire reproductive system; may relieve impotence

Sit with the soles of your feet together about a foot away from your body and let your knees fall toward the floor as far as possible. Grasp your ankles with both hands (A). Breathe in and straighten your spine, then breathe out and lean forward, pressing down on your thighs with your elbows (B). As you breathe in and straighten up, pull your feet in a little closer toward your body. Breathe out and bend forward again. Repeat once more for a total of three.

- Breathe deeply.
- Grab ankles with hands and press down with elbows.
- Don't strain. Hip and groin muscles take a fair amount of time to loosen up, so be patient. If you hurt the next day, you've done too much!

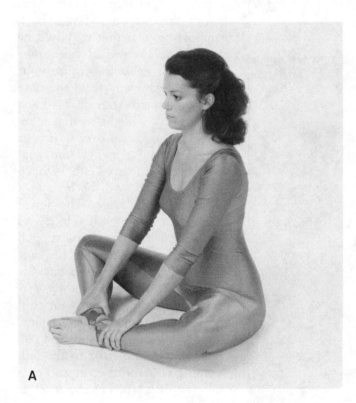

A

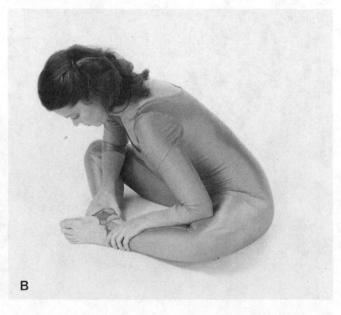

B

DIAMOND POSE I, II, III

(Shiva Shaktiasan)

Tones and strengthens entire nervous system
Strengthens and elongates sciatic nerve
Improves digestion
Strengthens and limbers hip joints
Limbers lower back

Place the soles of your feet together about a foot from your body. Lace your fingers around your toes (C). Your elbows will fall *outside* your legs in this exercise. Straighten your spine and breathe in deeply. Then breathe out and bend forward from the hips as far as you can without strain, letting your elbows fall outside your knees (D). Breathe in and straighten up. In the completed pose your big toes will be touching the center of your forehead. Repetitions: 3.

- Keep spine straight.
- Clasp toes.
- Elbows stay outside legs.

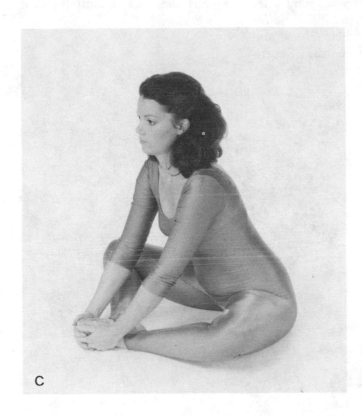

C

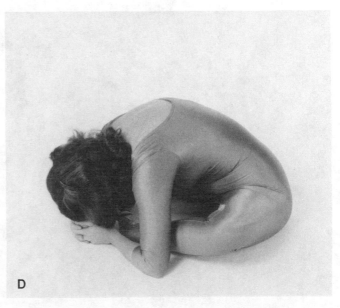

D

HERO POSE II, III
(Virasan)

Elongates spinal nerves, spinal cord and muscles of spinal column
Stretches lower back
Stretches and strengthens hips, knees and ankles
Elongates sciatic nerve and thigh muscles

Start with your right leg folded back and your left leg bent so that your left foot is against the inside of your right thigh (A), not underneath the leg. Place your hands on the floor above each knee, straighten your back, breathe in, then breathe out and bend forward, aiming your head at the midpoint between your knees. Breathe in and straighten up. With the next exhalation, bring your head in a little farther toward the right knee. On the third repetition, hold the downward position, breathing gently, and holding on to the outside of your right knee with your right hand (B). Hold for several seconds, then release and repeat on opposite side. Repetitions: 1 on each side.

When you become more limber, you may put your left foot on top of your right thigh (the whole foot, not just the toes), bringing your knees a little closer together (C). This very much increases the stretch on the hip joints and knees.

- Relax your hips and legs.
- Curl the toes around back of hip.

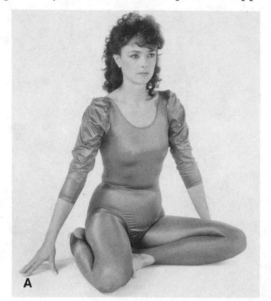

A

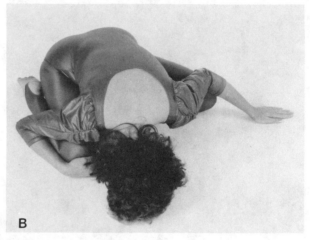

B

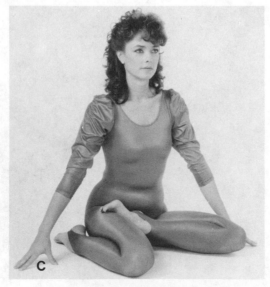

C

SIDE STRETCH III

Stretches side and intercostal muscles
Limbers vertebrae
Relieves tension in upper back and shoulders

Sit in a comfortable cross-legged position (see p. 132 for alternatives to the regular tailor position if you are limber enough) and sit straight with arms at your sides. Breathe normally throughout the exercise. Lean to the right on your right hand or elbow, and bring the other arm over your head in a plane with your body (A). Let the weight of your arm stretch the muscles along your left side and between your ribs. Bend your spine as far sideways as it will go without straining. Hang there for several seconds, then switch sides. Next, reverse the position of your feet and repeat.

- Keep upper arm in a plane with the body.
- Breathe normally
- Let the weight of your arm do the stretching.

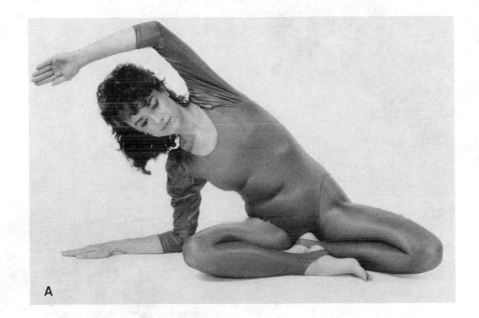

A

INTENSE FLOOR STRETCH I
(Uttihitasan)

Stretches muscles of torso and hips

Expands and stretches muscles of rib cage

Lines up vertebrae

Relieves back strain

Start by lying down with both arms resting on the floor over your head. First reach up with your right hand and push down with your right foot, keeping the foot flexed (A). Repeat with the left side. Then stretch opposite sides: left hand and right foot (B); right hand and left foot. This last opposite stretch is a swivel motion of the hips.

• Keep foot flexed.
• Breathe normally.

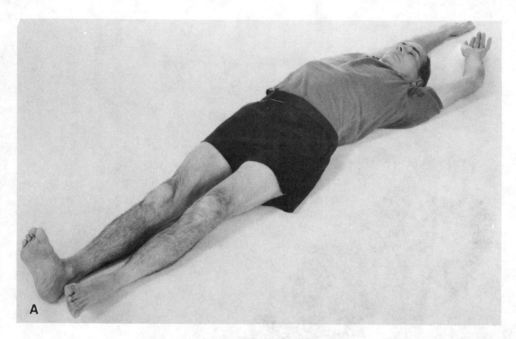

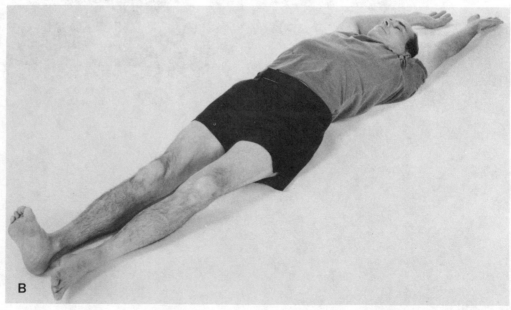

KNEE SQUEEZE I, II, III
(Pavanamuktasan)

Relieves gas, bloated sensation and heartburn in entire abdominal region; relieves constipation
Increases circulation in head and neck
Reduces body fat in abdomen and thighs
Relieves lower back tension
Strengthens abdominal muscles

Lie flat on your back with your arms at your sides (A). Begin to breathe in and raise your right knee to your chest. Make sure your lungs are all the way full, and wrap your arms around your knee. Hold your breath in and squeeze your knee to your chest (B). Exhale and slowly relax, straightening your leg (C). Repeat with your left leg. Repetitions: 3 on each side, alternating sides. Then rest a moment, breathing gently.

Now try the same exercise but lift both legs. In this variation it is important to breathe in *first*, then hold your breath in while you squeeze. If you try to breathe in and lift at the same time, you will not get a complete lungful of air because you will be tightening your stomach muscles to help you lift your legs. After a week or so of doing the double knee squeeze, you may add the following step: After you squeeze your knees to your chest, lift your forehead as far as possible between your knees (D). Then relax and breathe out. Repetitions: 3.

- Hold a full lungful of air in as you squeeze.
- In the double knee squeeze, breathe in first and hold your breath while you lift both knees to your chest.
- Hold the squeeze only a few seconds to start.

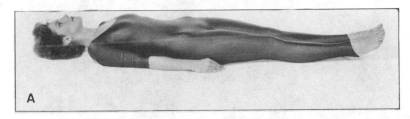

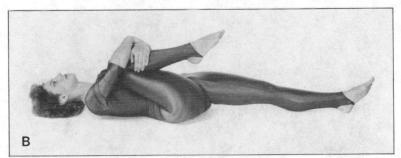

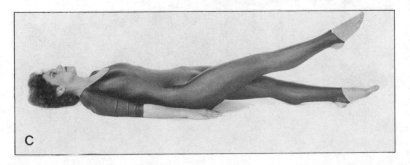

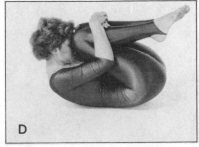

THE WALK II, III

*Reduces body fat from abdomen,
 hips, buttocks and thighs*
Strengthens legs
Helps relieve constipation
Strengthens lower back

Lie flat, arms at your sides, palms down. Bend your legs, then raise and straighten them so they are pointing toward the ceiling, at a 90-degree angle to your body. Breathing normally, start "walking" back and forth, keeping your legs straight and your feet flexed toward your face (A). Continue this motion for about thirty seconds, if you can; then bend your knees and slowly lower your legs to the floor.

• Keep legs straight.
• Keep feet flexed.
• Breathe normally.

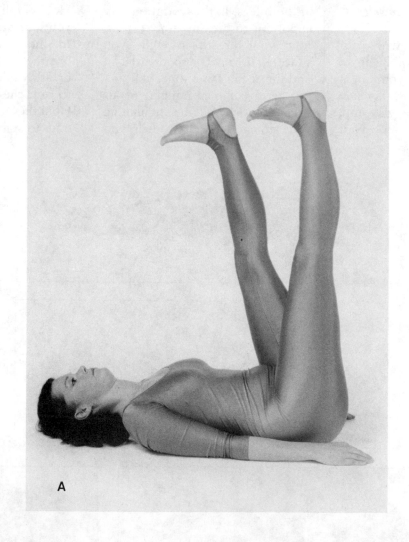

A

ALTERNATE TOE TOUCH II

(Supta Padangusthasan)

Tones, strengthens and promotes correct growth and development of bones and muscles in legs, helping relieve difficulties of sciatica and paralysis
Rejuvenates nerves and muscles in hips and pelvis
Strengthens lower back

Lie on your back with your arms on the floor. Breathe in and raise your left leg and left arm simultaneously (A). Keep your left foot flexed, your shoulders and head on the floor, and your right leg straight. If you cannot touch your toe, bring your arm and leg as close as possible. Hold for a moment, then relax and breathe out. Repetitions: 3 on each side.

Variation: With the same breath pattern, lift alternate arm and leg (B). Repetitions: 3 on each side.

- Keep shoulders and head on the floor.
- Keep both legs straight.
- Match breath with movement.

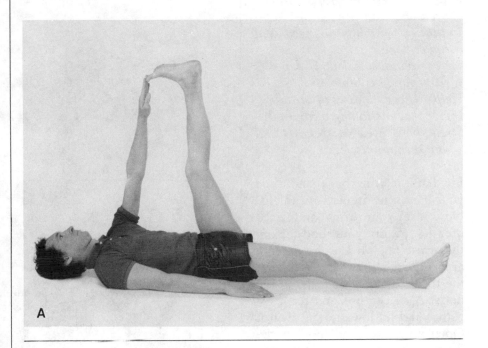

A

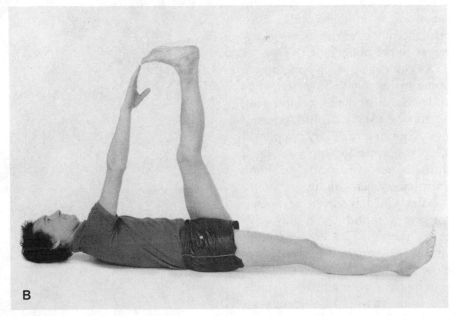

B

EASY FISH POSE II
(Matsyasan)

*Fully expands chest for improved
  breathing and circulation*
*Improves flexibility in neck and
  lower back*
*Helps remove calcium deposits
  from spinal column*
Helps relieve illnesses of throat
Improves functioning of thyroid
*Strengthens eyesight; tones facial
  and throat muscles*

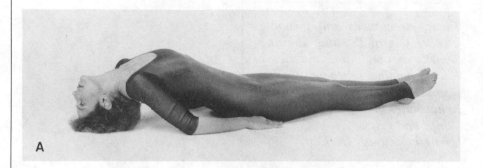

Lie flat on your back and slide
your hands just under your thighs.
Now use your arms and back
muscles to lift your body, from
the waist up, off the floor. Now
arch your back and neck so that
the top of your head rests on the
floor (A). Keep lips and teeth together and jut lower jaw forward.
Open your eyes and look at the
floor, breathing gently. Hold this
position several seconds, then
straighten spine as you gently
lower to the floor. Relax.

As you get up from lying down,
come up on one elbow first, then
slide the other hand behind you,
as shown (B), and push yourself
up. This intermediary step will
keep you from tensing your back
muscles and possibly straining
your back when you lift.

After you have been practicing
for several months, you may wish
to try the Full Fish Pose. Start by
sitting between your feet, knees as
close together as possible, then
lean back on your elbows. Usually
this is as far as most students can
go until the thigh and groin muscles loosen up more. Keep practicing this intermediary step and
eventually you will be able to take
the full position as shown (C).

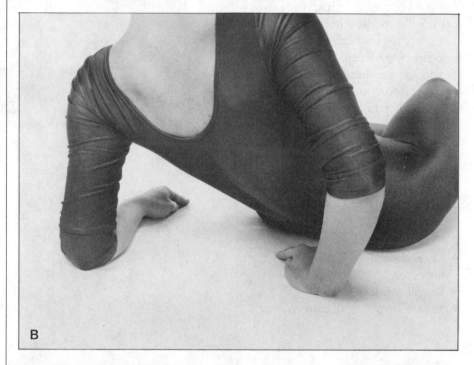

- Keep lips and teeth together.
- Keep eyes open.
- Let breath relax into the belly.

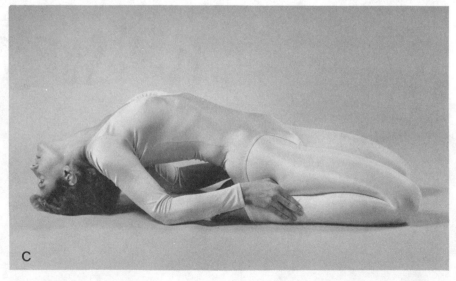

PELVIC TWIST I
Jathara Parivarthanasan)

Improves activity and functioning of liver, spleen, pancreas, stomach, kidneys and intestines
Reduces excess fat from waist
Strengthens lower back and hips

Do not do this exercise if you have lower back problems. Lie on your back with your arms straight out to the sides, palms down. Lift your legs and feet off the floor as if you were going to do a double knee squeeze (A). This is your starting position. Breathe in as you slowly swing your legs toward the floor to the right, keeping your knees bent and feet off the floor (B). If you wish (if you do not have neck problems), you may turn your head the opposite way to relieve any upper back tension that may accumulate as you twist. Breathe out and slowly raise your legs back up to the starting position. Then breathe in and lower to the left. Breathe out and return to the center. Be sure to keep your shoulders and arms on the floor at all times. Repetitions: 3 on each side.

After doing this exercise for several weeks, you may move on to a more difficult variation. Keep the same starting position, but as you lower your legs to the side, breathing in, straighten them so that they are parallel to your outstretched arm (C). Repetitions: 3 on each side.

- Keep shoulders and arms on the floor.
- Breathe deeply and slowly, matching breath with movement.

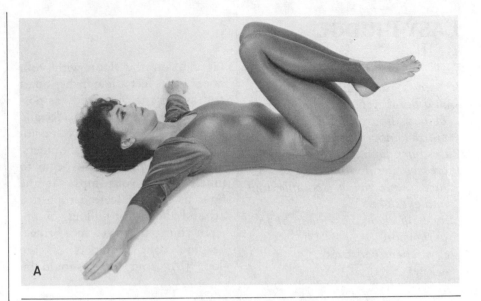

A

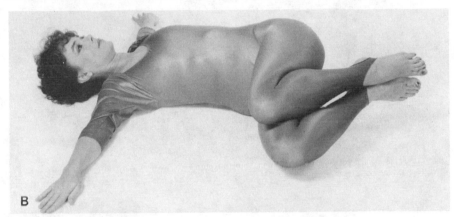

B

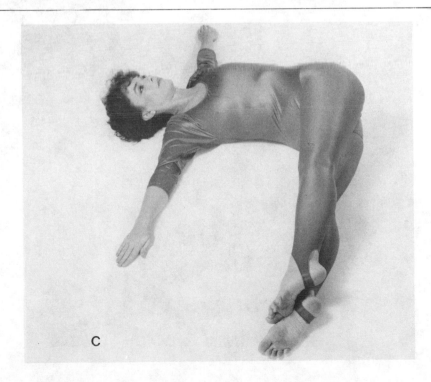

C

EASY BRIDGE I, II, III

Improves functioning of thyroid and parathyroid glands, thereby helping improve functioning of entire endocrine system

Eases back pain and fatigue

Increases circulation to head and face, improving complexion and eyesight

May help in management of hypertension

Helps relieve bedsores

Lie flat on the floor with your knees bent, feet a few inches apart and as close to your body as possible. Place arms at your sides and palms down (A). Breathe out completely, and relax your shoulders, neck and head. As you begin to inhale, raise your hips off the floor as if there were a rope tied around your waist pulling you up. Arch your back into a nice bridge, keeping your shoulders on the floor (B). Your lungs should be filled in the arched position. Now breathe out and slowly lower your hips to the floor. Be sure not to turn your head in this position. Repetitions: 3. (If you can reach your ankles easily, you may do this exercise holding on to your ankles as shown (C).)

- Keep shoulders and neck relaxed.
- Place feet as close to body as possible.

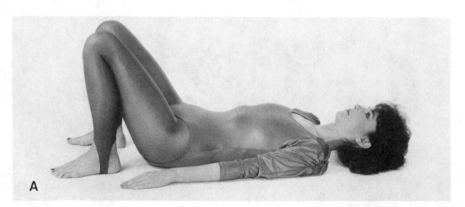

A

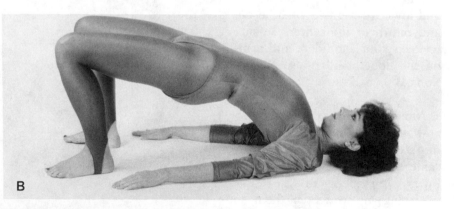

B

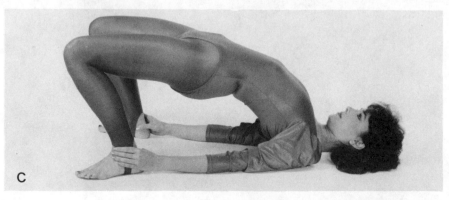

C

EASY SIT-UP II, III

Strengthens abdominal muscles and upper back
Relieves stomach and breath tension
Massages internal organs

Lie on your back with your knees bent and your feet a comfortable distance apart. Straighten your arms and place your fingers on your thighs (they should be a few inches down from your knees (A).) Now breathe in until your lungs are about one-half full, and hold your breath in as you lift your head and upper body, sliding your hands up to your knees (B). Hold a moment at the top, and relax and breathe out. Repetitions: 3.

• Keep arms straight.
• Hold breath in as you lift.

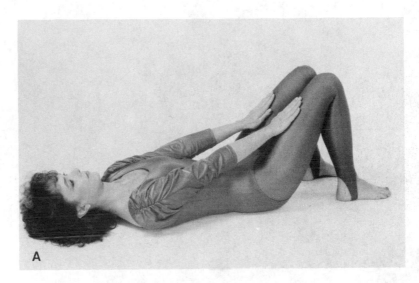

A

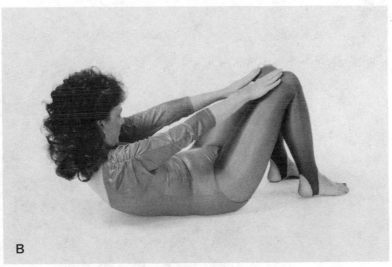

B

NECK CURL II, III

Strengthens stomach and upper back

Relieves breath and stomach tension

Similar to the Easy Sit-up, this exercise is a little easier on the neck for students with neck problems. Lie on your back with your knees up, feet a comfortable distance apart. Place your hands on your upper back and shoulders, spreading your fingers to support your neck (A). An alternate position is to cross your arms on your chest, holding opposite shoulders. Breathe in to about one-half capacity, then hold your breath in and lift, using your back and stomach muscles (B). Do not strain. Relax and breathe out. Repetitions: 3.

• Hold breath in while lifting.
• Support your neck.

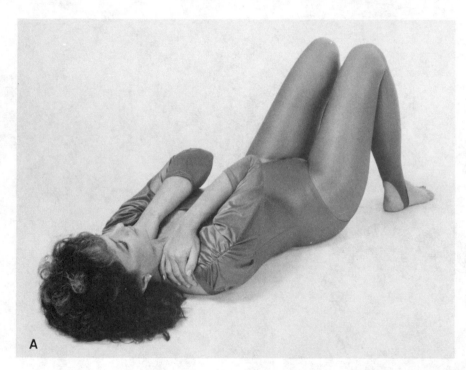

A

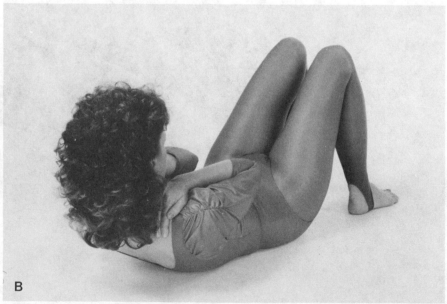

B

BIG SIT-UP II, III
(Supta Padangusthasan)

*Strengthens abdominal viscera
and all abdominal and thigh
muscles*

Improves balance and concentration

Strengthens legs

Relieves constipation and difficulties of urinary tract

This is the most challenging of the sit-up exercises. Lie flat on your back with arms on the floor overhead (A). Breathe in to about half capacity, hold your breath in and raise both arms and legs simultaneously. Balancing on the end of your spine, reach up to touch your toes (B). Hold for a moment if you can. Then lower and breathe out. Repetitions: 3 to 6.

- Keep legs straight.
- Hold breath in as you raise.
- Breathe shallowly.

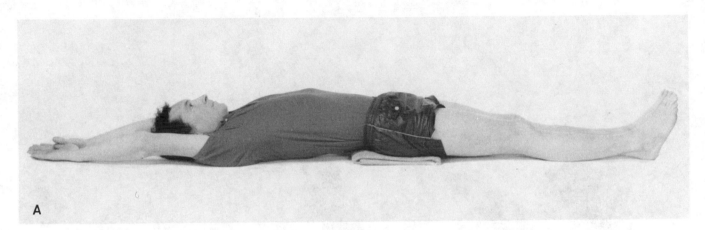

A

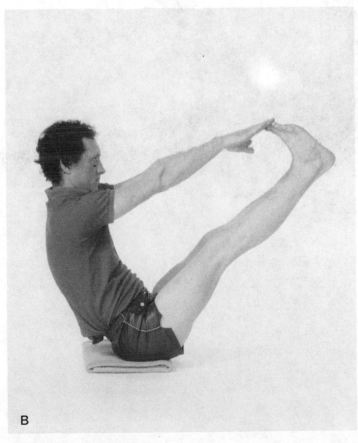

B

ALTERNATE BIG SIT-UP III

Strengthens transverse abdominal muscles

Strengthens lower back and shoulders

Limbers and strengthens hip joints

Lie on your back with arms at your side. Breathe in to about one-half capacity, hold your breath in, then raise your left arm, your torso and your right leg, leaning on your right elbow as shown (A). Keep your foot flexed. Touch your toes if possible, then breathe out and return to starting position. Repetitions: 3 to 6 each side, alternating.

- Keep legs and arms straight.
- Hold breath in as you lift.
- Lean on opposite elbow for support.

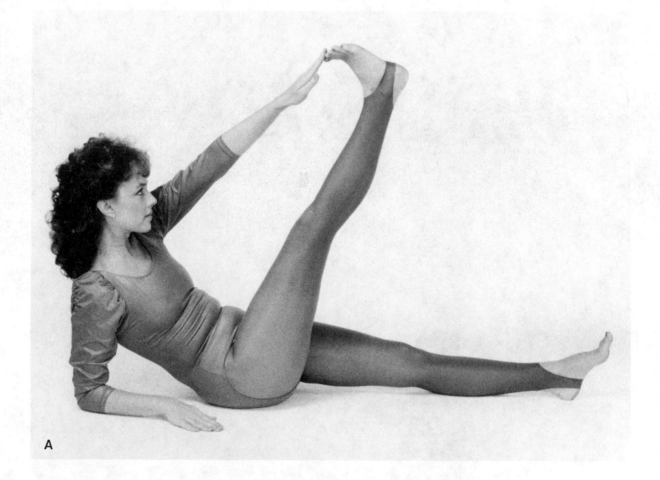

A

THE ROLL I

Helps make spine flexible and limber in preparation for Shoulder Stand

Sit with knees drawn up to your chest, head down, back rounded and arms clasped around your knees (A). Holding this position, roll backward on your spine (B) then roll up to a seated position. Be sure to give yourself enough momentum. If you find that your back is too stiff to stay rounded, you can place your hands on the floor next to your body and push off. Roll back and forth several times. Practice this exercise for a few weeks before attempting the Shoulder Stand.

- Keep your chin tucked.
- Round your back as much as possible.

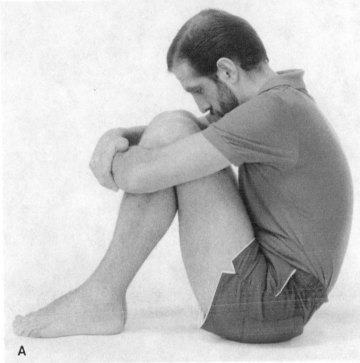

A

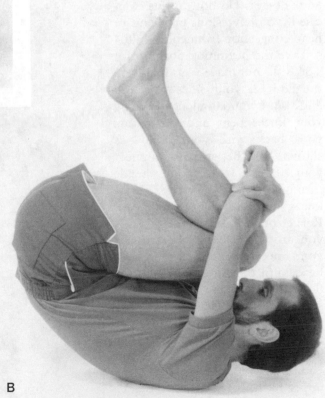

B

SHOULDER STAND
I, II, III
(Sarvangasan)

Tones the entire endocrine system through stimulation of thyroid and parathyroid glands

Enhances function of all vital organs

May improve reproductive function

Helps relieve many respiratory difficulties

Improves eyesight

Relieves tension on heart and lungs

Relaxes entire nervous system

Relieves constipation and may help epilepsy

Removes fatigue and makes mind bright and clear

Helps yeast infections

This pose should not be done by people with high blood pressure, heart disease or neck problems without specific permission from your doctor. Do not do this exercise if you have sinus problems or head congestion from cold or flu.

Take the beginning position for The Roll, but place your hands on the floor at your sides (A). Roll back onto your shoulders, keeping your knees bent and supporting your back with your hands as shown (B). Be sure to support your back with your hands throughout the exercise. Your knees should touch your forehead. Relax your shoulders and head. If you are comfortable, start to lift your knees away from your forehead until they are parallel to the floor (C). Then continue to straighten your legs while supporting your back with your hands (D). First straighten your legs at an angle; in this position your weight will be more on your upper back, between the shoulder

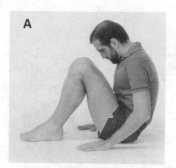

A

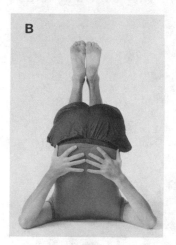

B

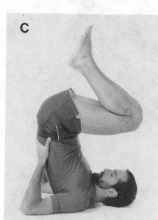

C

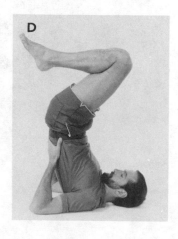

D

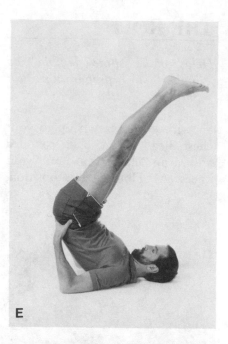

E

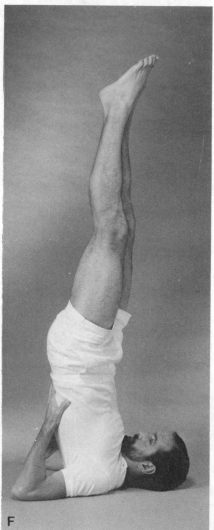

F

blades, than on your neck (E). Practice this Half Shoulder Stand for several days before going on to the completed pose.

When you go to the completed pose (F), try to straighten your legs so that they are upright. Keep feet relaxed, not pointed. You will notice that you can straighten your body more by bringing your hands farther down your back toward the floor and pressing gently while supporting. Your weight is now on the back of your neck. Hold the position, breathing gently, for several seconds. Fix your gaze on the space between your big toes; your feet should be touching. If your eyes get tired, close them for a moment. In the beginning, hold this pose for only 10 to 15 seconds. Do not turn your head.

To come out of the position safely, bend your knees and bring them to your forehead, cross your ankles and gently roll forward all the way, so that your legs fall apart into a cross-legged position and your head is bent forward. This is to prevent faintness from having the blood rush out of your head too quickly. Remain in this position for several seconds.

If you have difficulty lifting your legs, you may lack strength in your arms and back. If so, practice pushing off from a chair (G) or a wall (H) until your back and arms develop the proper supportive strength.

- Support your back at all times.
- Straighten your legs slowly.
- Breathe normally.
- Relax as much as possible.

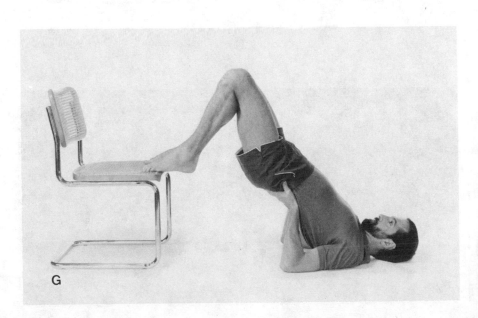

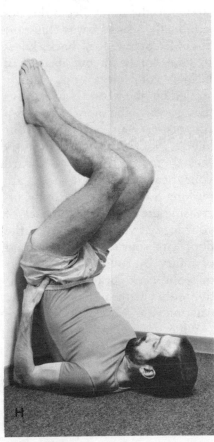

PLOW POSE I, II, III
(Halasan)

Stimulates the thyroid and para-thyroid glands, improving functioning of entire endocrine system

Gives a complete stretch to spinal cord, nerves and muscles, and muscles and nerves of legs

Relieves constipation and lumbago, and helps muscular rheumatism

Reduces body fat

Relieves enlargement of liver and spleen

Improves posture and suppleness of spine by preventing ossification of vertebrae

Stretches arteries and veins, making them more supple, elastic and strong

The Plow Pose intensifies the stretch to the spine. Begin this position the same way as the Shoulder Stand. Roll back, knees to your forehead, but instead of lifting your legs up, slowly straighten them and lower your toes toward the floor (A). Keep supporting your back with your hands. Notice that your toes are tucked under, pointing toward your head, and your heels are pushing away from your body, increasing the stretch on the back of your legs. If you cannot reach the floor with your toes and are afraid of injury by rolling back too far on your neck, practice this position either with a chair (B) or by walking your feet down the wall.

When you get into position, you can release the back support and straighten your arms out, palms down (C). Hold the position for several seconds, breathing gently. Be sure not to do this position or the Shoulder Stand if you have a

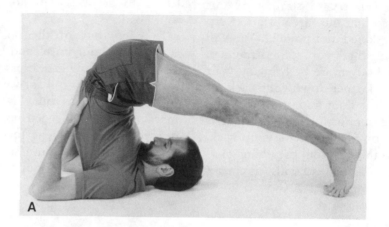

A

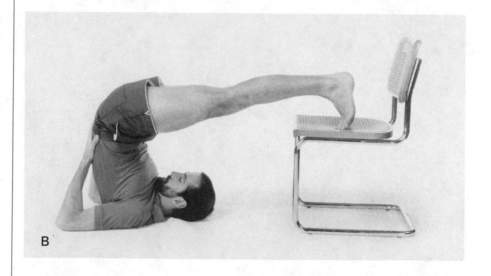

B

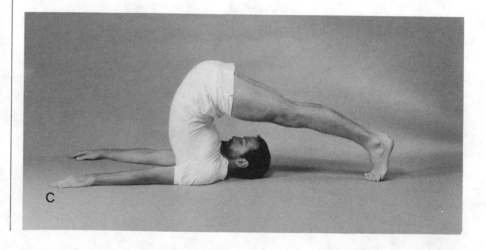

C

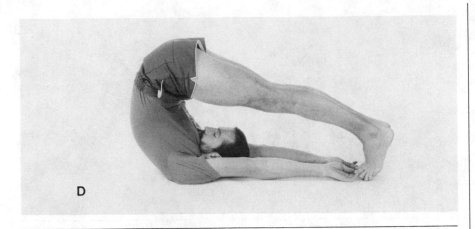

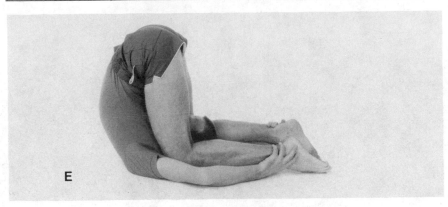

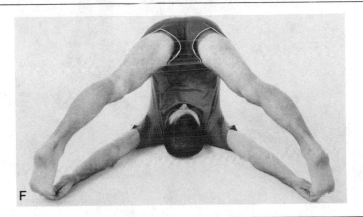

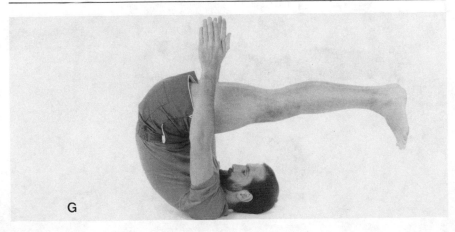

head cold or nasal congestion. If you notice headaches after doing this exercise, that should indicate that you are putting too much strain on the muscles and nerves, especially in the back of your neck, and you should proceed more cautiously.

When you have gained flexibility, stamina and assurance in this practice, you may try some of the variations. Bring your arms around so that you grasp your big toes (D). Press your heels toward the floor as far as possible. Next, lower your knees so that they rest on the floor next to your ears. Hold onto your feet with both hands (E). Now straighten your legs, grab your big toes again and spread your legs as far as possible (F). Bring your legs back together, lift them off the floor until you are balanced, then straighten your arms slowly up toward the ceiling, resting on your shoulders and neck (G). This variation brings a beautiful complexion and clarity of mind.

To come out of the Plow Pose, bring your knees to your forehead, support your back with your hands and slowly roll forward, bending your head over crossed legs as you did after the Shoulder Stand. Always use your common sense when practicing these asans; never strain past your physical limitations. Yoga is a nonviolent practice, especially with regard to your own body.

- Keep legs straight and shoulders relaxed.
- Breathe gently.
- Do not exceed your limits.

EASY PLOW BREATH
III

Relieves tension in breath and midsection
Strengthens abdominal, lower back and leg muscles
Stimulates functioning of internal organs

Start on your back, with bent knees, arms at your sides, palms down (A). Breathe in fully, then breathe out as you straighten your legs (B) and bring them over your head until they are several inches above the floor (C). You will need to give yourself some momentum, using your arms, to initially lift your legs up and over. Notice that the action of bringing your legs over your head has the effect of naturally pushing your breath out in an exhalation. Now start to inhale and lower your legs; first lower them straight until your hips touch the floor, then bend your legs and bring your feet back down to the floor. Your breath should be completely in at this point. Immediately start to breathe out and bring your legs up straight again and over your head, repeating the first movement with the exhalation. Repetitions: 3 to 6.

- Use arms only to augment back muscles.
- Keep legs straight when lifting over head.
- Breathe out when legs go over head; breathe in when legs come back down to the floor.

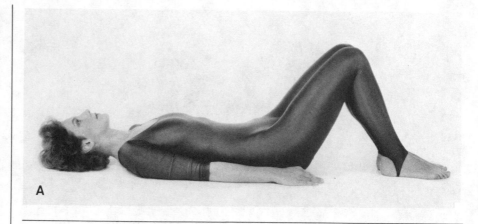

A

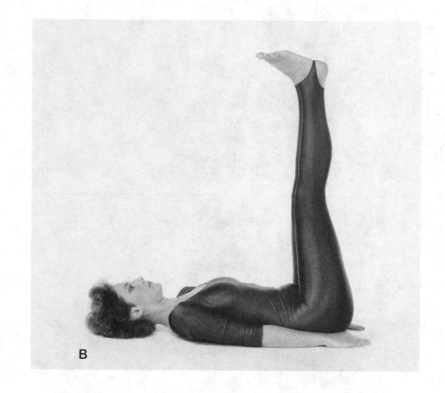

B

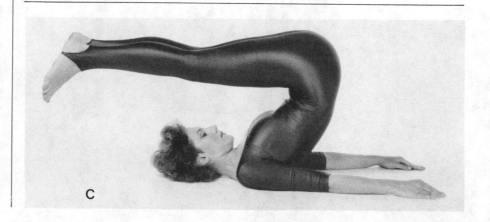

C

PLOW BREATH III

Relieves tension in breath and midsection
Strengthens abdominal, lower back and leg muscles
Stimulates functioning of internal organs

Start lying on your back with arms at your sides, palms down (A). Breathe in, hold your breath in and lift your legs up, keeping them straight (B). As your legs reach the point where they are straight up (but without stopping the momentum of your legs), start breathing out. The impetus of your legs going over your head will force the breath out further. Continue lowering your legs until they touch the floor over your head, as in the Plow Pose (C). Now lift them back up and start breathing in as you lift your legs up and back down straight. Try not to touch the floor with your heels but lift them back up in another repetition of the exercise right away. Repetitions: 3 to 6.

- Keep legs straight.
- Breathe out as legs go over your head; breathe in as they come back down to the floor.
- Try to let the motion of your body control your breath.

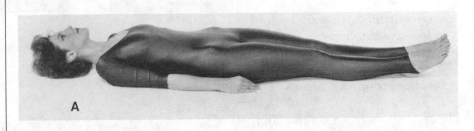

A

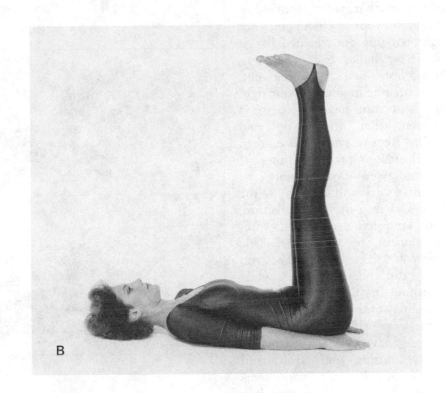

B

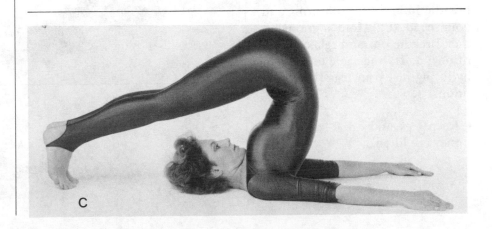

C

BACK STRENGTHENERS I, II

Strengthens all back muscles and entire spinal column

Increases abdominal pressure, which improves digestion and functioning of vital organs

Lie on your stomach on the floor, with arms outstretched in front (A). Bend your left arm at the elbow so that your forehead is resting on your left hand and your right remains outstretched (B). If you have upper back problems, bend *both* arms. Breathe out. Now breathe in and lift your right arm and your head. Hold for a moment, then breathe out and lower. Repeat twice more, then switch sides and repeat 3 times.

After a few days of practicing the first variation, go on to the next. Get into the same position, with your left arm folded, forehead resting on your hand. This time you will raise your right arm, your head and your left leg while breathing in (C). Later, you can straighten both arms (D). Repetitions: 3 each side, alternating.

The final back strengtheners involve lifting the arms and legs separately. Start with arms outstretched in front, forehead to the floor. Breathe out. Now breathe in and lift both arms and your head (E). Hold a moment, then breathe out and relax. Repetitions: 3. Try the same movement by lifting just your legs (F). Repetitions: 3.

• Keep legs and arms straight as they are lifted.

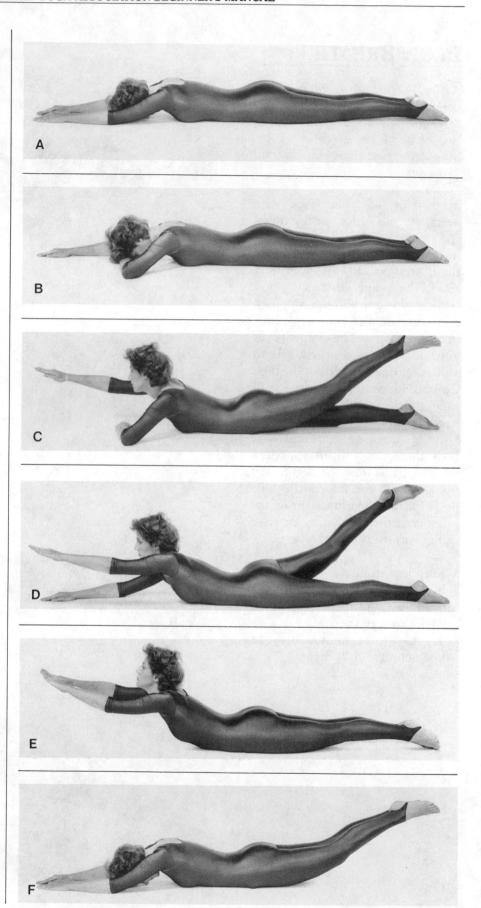

BOAT POSE I, II
(Poorva Navasan)

Strengthens all back muscles and entire spinal column

Increases abdominal pressure, which improves digestion and functioning of vital organs

Lie on your stomach, forehead to the floor, arms outstretched in front (A). Breathe out completely. Then breathe in to one-half to two-thirds capacity, hold your breath in and lift your arms, head and legs as high as possible (B). Look up, hold for a moment, then breathe out and relax. Breathing in and holding your breath in before you lift will help prevent getting a cramp in the diaphragm from trying to breathe and lift at the same time, using your abdominal muscles. Repetitions: 3.

- Keep legs and arms straight.
- Hold breath in as you lift.

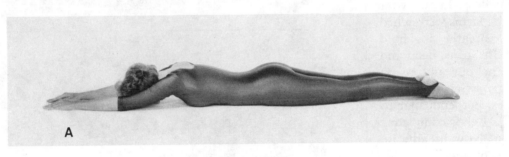

A

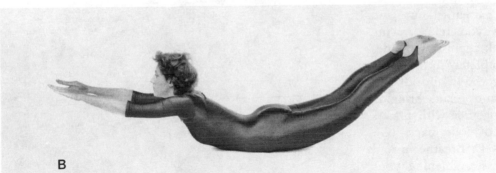

B

AIRPLANE SERIES
II

Strengthens entire back and spinal column

Improves functioning of vital organs

Limbers spinal column and shoulder joints

Strengthens arms, shoulders, hips and thighs

Expands rib cage, improving breathing

This is a more challenging series to attempt after you have become proficient with the Back Strengtheners and Boat Pose. Lie on your stomach with arms stretched overhead (A). Breathe in, hold breath in and lift: arms, head and legs (B). Breathe out and relax, but as you relax, swing your arms out to the sides, perpendicular to your body (C). Relax completely in this position. Now breathe in, hold the breath in and lift in this position (D); breathe out and relax, but as you relax, swing your arms back against your sides (E). Relax completely in this position. Now breathe in and lift (F); breathe out and relax, bringing your hands together with fingers clasped behind your back (G). Relax completely. Breathe in and lift up again, straightening your arms as much as possible and lifting them up away from your back (H). Breathe out and relax, bending your knees and holding on to your toes, feet or ankles (I). Relax completely. Now breathe in and lift up for the fifth in the series, the Bow Pose (J) and then breathe out and relax, arms to your sides. Rest for several seconds, until your breath returns to normal and your body is completely relaxed.

When you have practiced these five positions for several days, you

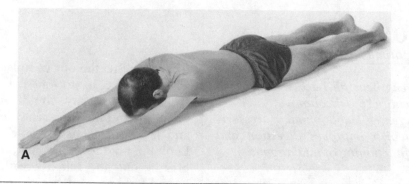

A

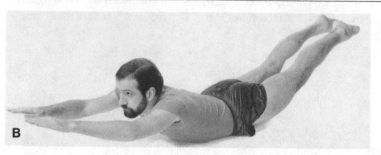

B

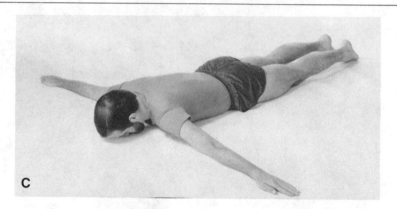

C

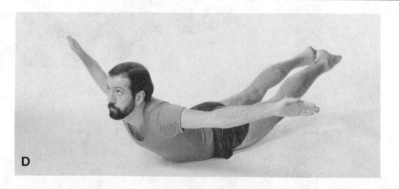

D

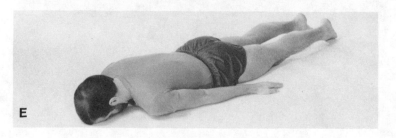

E

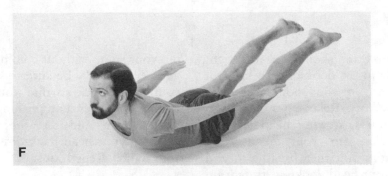

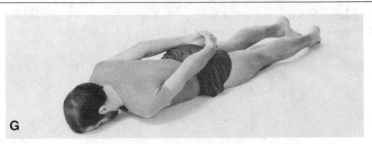

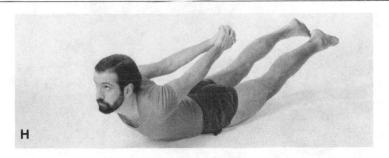

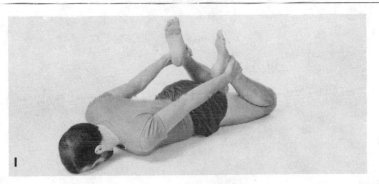

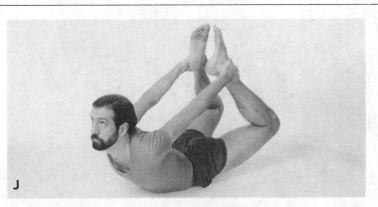

can add repetitions by reversing direction. When you reach the Bow Pose, do it twice, then relax into the hands-clasped position, then lift and relax with arms at sides, and so on back up to the beginning Boat Pose with arms out in front. Repetitions: 1 to 5 sequences.

- Keep arms and legs straight.
- Breathe in and hold breath in as you lift.
- Relax completely between each lift.

EASY COBRA POSE I

Limbers and straightens spinal column and back muscles
Strengthens upper back and shoulders
Prepares for Cobra Pose

Lie on your stomach and come up on your elbows with hands clasped in front of you. Your upper arms should be at a right angle to the floor, directly straight down from your shoulder joint to the elbow. Relax your head and shoulders, so your head rests on or close to your hands (A). Breathe out, then breathe in and lift your head, looking straight up at the ceiling. Stretch up and back a little, stretching and compressing your spine without coming off your elbows (B). Be sure to relax your lower back so that you are curling up rather than pushing up. Then relax and breathe out, bringing your head back down to your hands. Repetitions: 3.

• Keep elbows on the floor.
• Relax lower back.

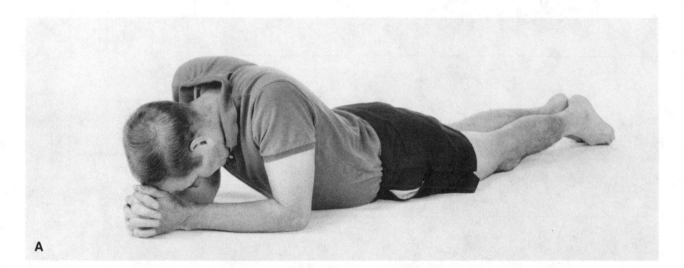

A

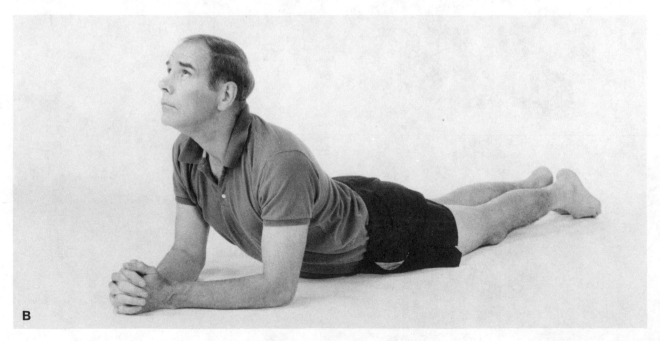

B

COBRA POSE I, II, III

(Bhujangasan)

Improves functioning of intestines
Increases body heat
Strengthens back muscles and limbers spinal column
Stimulates proper functioning of reproductive system
Increases overall body strength
Strengthens eyesight

Lie on your stomach with toes together, forehead on the floor and palms down next to your armpits (A). Your elbows will be up in the air. Begin to breathe in and raise just your head, looking straight up at all times. Continue to lift your chest, then your stomach, curling your spine rather than pushing with your arms (B and C). Be sure not to lift so high that your hip bones come off the floor. Try to use mostly your back muscles to lift rather than your arms, although your arms are available for balance and support. Do not lift high enough to be able to straighten your arms. Keep your lips and teeth together, and jut your jaw forward slightly to tense the throat muscles. Hold the position for a moment, then start to breathe out and uncurl slowly, keeping your head back until the very last. Your stomach touches first, then your chest and finally your head, tucking it forward so the forehead rests against the floor. Then relax until your breath returns to normal. This is a very powerful exercise that brings energy to all parts of the body and especially equalizes the two halves of the body. Repetitions: 3.

- Curl your spine using your back muscles rather than by pushing up with your arms.
- Your head should come up first and down last.
- Hip bones must stay on the floor.

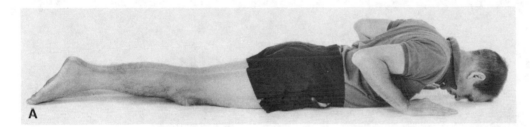

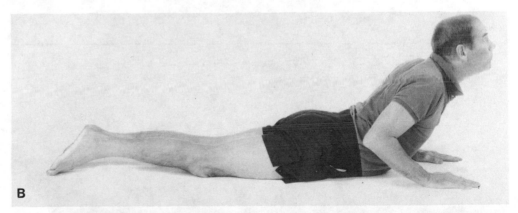

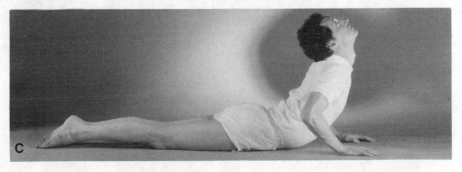

BOW POSE I, II
(Dhanurasan)

Relieves chronic constipation
Improves functioning of liver, kidneys, spleen, stomach and intestines
Strengthens the back and thighs
Aligns vertebrae properly
Increases vigor and vitality

Lie flat on your stomach with your forehead on the floor, and bend your legs at the knees. Reach back and grasp both feet or ankles (A). Now, breathe in deeply, hold your breath in and raise yourself up, pulling your feet up and away from your body for a maximum stretch to the spine (B). Look up, and keep your lips and teeth together. Hold for a moment, then breathe out and lower yourself to the floor. Repetitions: 3

- Keep eyes open, looking up.
- Lift feet up and away from your body.
- Hold breath in as you lift.

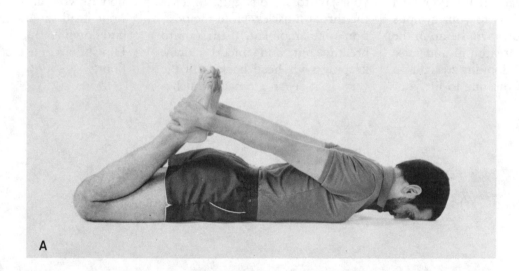

A

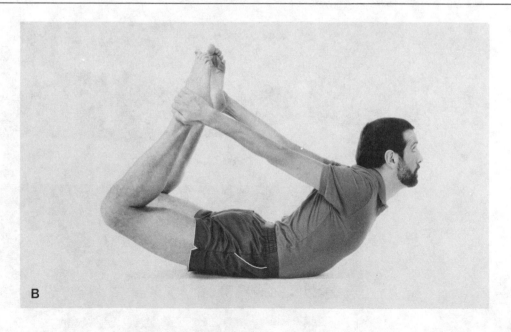

B

SUN SALUTATION II, III

(Surya Namaskar)

*Stimulates circulation throughout
  entire body*
Strengthens breathing muscles
Limbers spine in both directions
*Stretches and strengthens hip and
  thigh muscles*

This is an important sequence that combines the stretching and strengthening functions of several major asans. Before trying this exercise, you should have begun the Course Two routine and should be fairly proficient in the Standing Sun Pose, Cobra Pose, Thigh Stretch and Cobra V-Raise. It is named the Sun Salutation because it is health-giving, like the sun, and because the sequence of movements represents the passage of the sun through the day and through the year.

Start in a standing position with palms together in the traditional greeting of India: *"Namaste"* (A). Breathe in and raise your arms in a wide circle overhead (B), picturing your arms bringing the sun up with the movement. Stretch at the

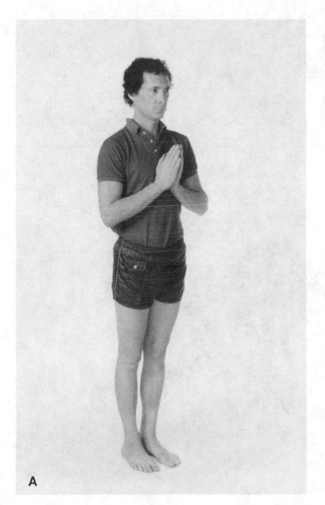

A

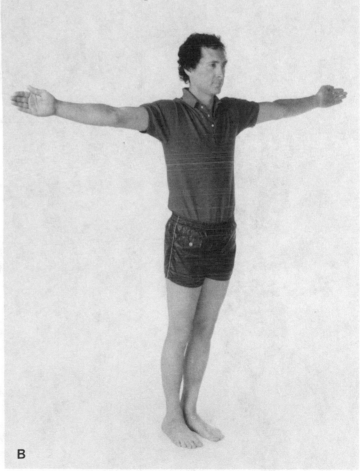

B

top and look up at your hands (C). Then breathe out and bend from the hips, keeping your head between your arms (D). Bend as far forward as possible, grasp your ankles and pull your upper body toward your legs with your breath held out (E).

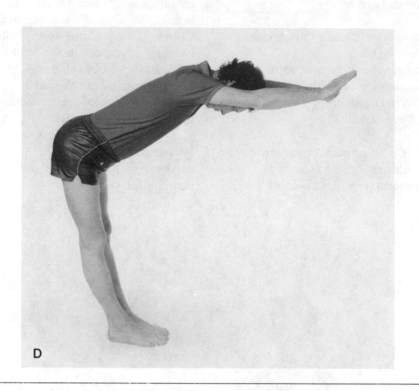

D

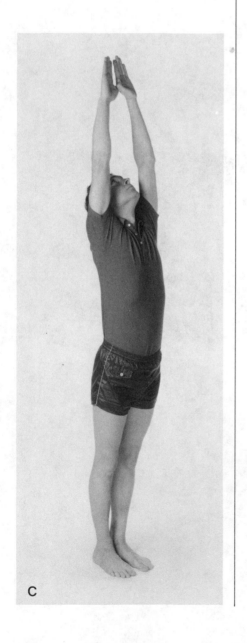

C

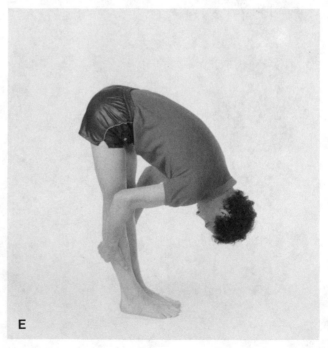

E

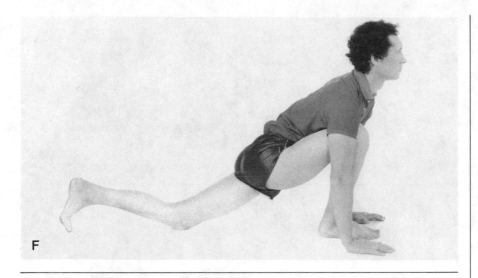

F

Now start to breathe in as you lunge forward with your right foot into position as if you were going to do the Thigh Stretch (F). Continue breathing in and raise your arms overhead, arching your back and pushing your hips forward as you feel the stretch in your thighs (G). Look up. In the beginning keep your back knee on the floor, but after a few weeks of practice try holding the knee up.

Now hold your breath in and come to a Plank Pose, arms straight and body on a plane (H).

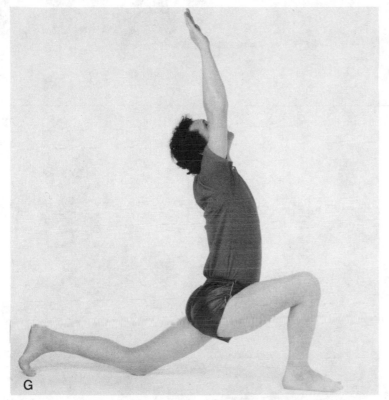

G

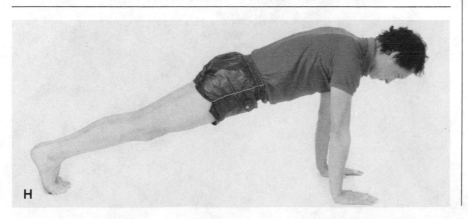

H

Next, come down so that your knees, chest and chin are touching the floor, a zigzag position (I).

Breathe out and flatten your body, keeping your hands next to your shoulders (J).

Breathe in and arch up into a Cobra Pose (K).

Tuck your toes under and breathe out, pushing your hips up into a V-raise (L).

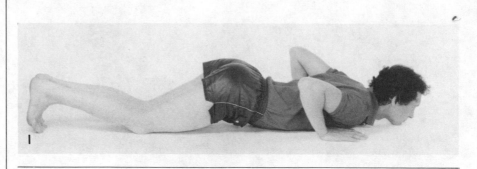

I

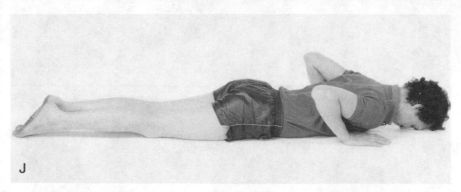

J

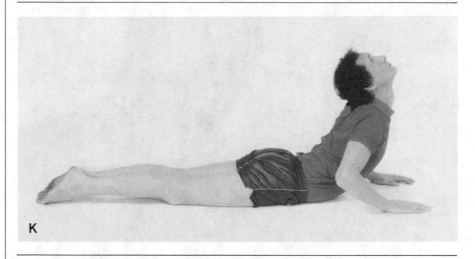

K

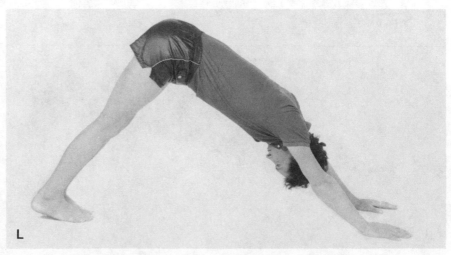

L

Now start to breathe in and lunge forward with the left foot into position as if for the Thigh Stretch (M). Continue breathing in while you raise your arms in a wide circle overhead and look up (N).

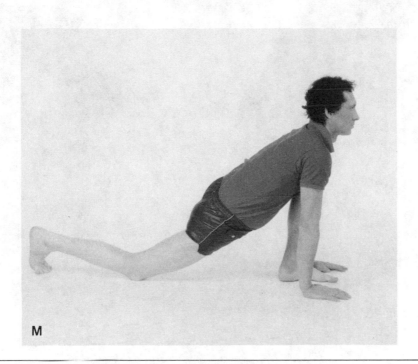

M

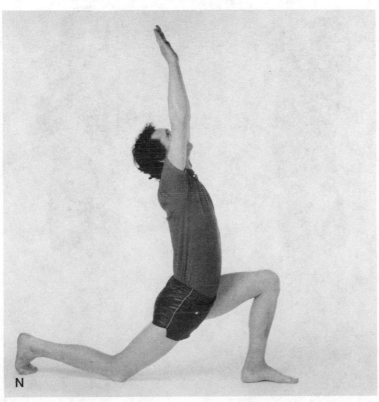

N

Then breathe out, bring your back leg forward and grasp your legs as in the bottom of the Standing Sun Pose (O). Breathe in and begin to stand up, bringing your arms in a wide circle to the sides (P) and overhead, lock thumbs, and look up at your hands (Q). Then breathe out, lower your arms to the sides, and bring them back to the salutation position, palms together (R). Repetitions: 3 to 5.

- Breathe deeply and coordinate breathing with movement.
- Do not strain.

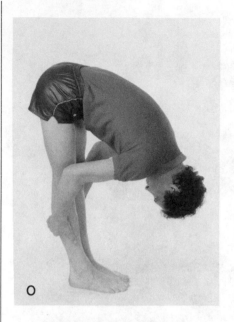

O

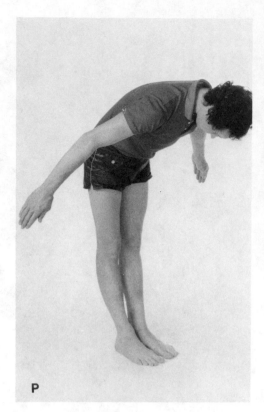

P

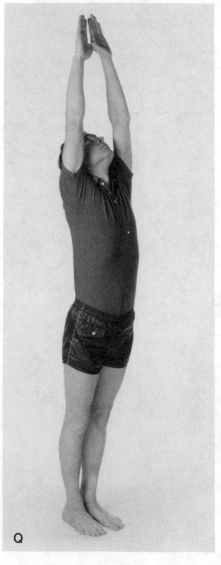

Q

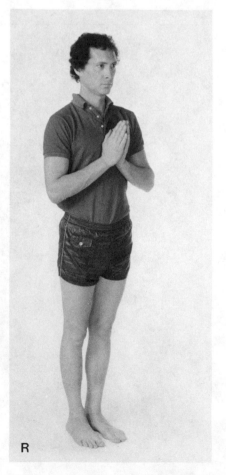

R

CHAPTER 5
BREATHING (PRANAYAMA)

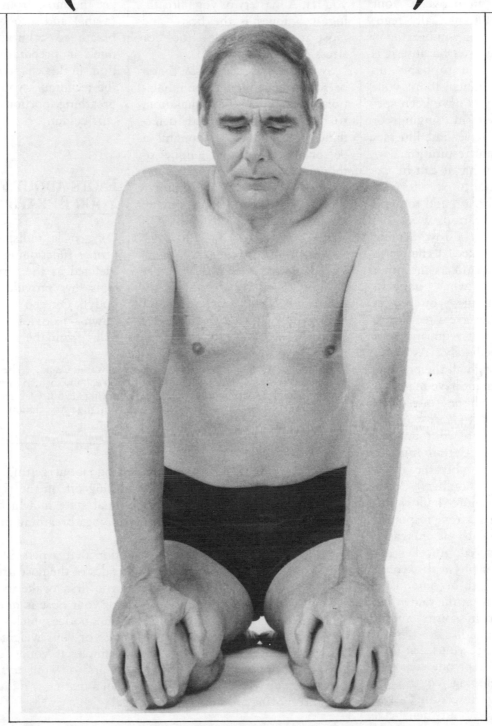

BREATHING TECHNIQUES

Breathing is probably the most important thing you do in life; in fact, without breath, you wouldn't be able to do anything at all!

Breath is with you from the moment you are born until the instant you die. In between, your body usually automatically regulates how much air you breathe in and breathe out. Yet because it is so automatic, you probably do not think very much about your breath, unless you have been specifically trained in singing or sports or you have had illnesses that affected your respiration.

Yogis believe that it can be extremely beneficial to pay more attention to the breath and to learn to control it in various ways. Because the breath, body and mind are so closely linked, a change in one immediately affects the other two. Consider what happens when, for example, you are at work and you receive a terse message from the boss requiring your presence immediately. As your mind goes through all the possible mistakes you might have made, or the praise you hope to receive, your breath and body respond to the emotional state your imaginings have elicited. Certain muscles become tense (notably the stomach, face and shoulders); your breath becomes more shallow and short; and other stress responses in your body, such as increased pulse, are triggered. Another example: vigorous physical exercise causes breathing to become faster and deeper, while at the same time effecting a lift in spirits and a calming of the mind.

In yoga practice you learn how to take this concept one step further. By developing control of your breathing in certain ways, you can bring about beneficial changes in your body and mind. Remember a parent or teacher telling you, when you were upset, to "sit down and take a deep breath and you'll feel better"? It really does work! In yoga you learn how to do it systematically, so that results happen each time you try. A mastery of yoga breathing techniques is the best—and most readily available—tool for stress reduction.

Swami Rama used to say that a person has one thought on inhalation and another on exhalation, so that the rate of breath determines the number of thoughts a person has.* A greater number of thoughts (a faster breathing rate) thus results in lower concentration because there are so many thoughts going on:

*As the numbers of ideas conceived by the mind increases, their power of fulfillment decreases; conversely, the fewer ideas the mind lingers over for a comparatively longer time, the greater their power of fulfillment, because these ideas are backed by the force of the mind. This force is called willpower.**

In your beginning yoga practice, you will learn how to use correct breath patterns in order to get the most from your exercises (asans) and also how to use the breath to calm and quiet your mind in preparation for meditation. In this chapter you will learn the techniques you'll need for the breathing portion of your yoga curriculum.

FACTS ABOUT YOGA AND YOUR BREATH

Oxygen is indispensable to the proper functioning of metabolism (defined as the physiological systems that provide energy for the body). Oxygen is used to break down—to oxidize—nutrient particles from the food we eat into

---

*For amplification of this theory, refer to the books listed in Suggested Reading for this chapter, particularly Light on Pranayama, by Iyengar.

*Swami Rama, "The World, a Fancy Tree," in Yoga in America, Vol. IV:1, Spring, 1980. Cleveland, Ohio: American Yoga Association.

Are you familiar with the saying about getting up on the wrong side of the bed or starting off on the right foot in reference to the mental or emotional state in which a person begins his day? There is a theory in yoga breathing practice that pertains to this old saying.

This theory is based on the notion that a person feels more balanced, more stable, when both sides of the nose are functioning approximately equally. When you first awake in the morning, you may notice that one side of your nose is more stopped up than the other. Before you stand up, notice which side is clear. Then put your foot down with most of your weight for a few seconds *first* on that side. For example, if your right side is stuffed up, put your weight down first on your *left* foot. The stuffed up (right) side will clear up in a matter of minutes as you start moving around. Try it and see!

simpler and more absorbable forms. Carbon dioxide and other waste products, along with a release of energy, are the end products of this process. The energy that is produced is what allows our muscles and other tissues to perform the work that we demand of them. Even the brain's tissues require oxygen for thinking, remembering and other mental processes. In fact, the brain requires about three times as much oxygen as the rest of the body. Lack of oxygen nourishment can contribute to sluggishness, fatigue, confusion, loss of memory and disorientation.

Yoga practice increases oxygen flow to the brain and body in several ways. First it *increases the vital capacity* of the lungs, that is, the volume of air that you are able to inhale. Studies have shown that yoga training actually increases vital capacity over a period of several months.* This does not mean that the lungs increase in size but rather that through exercise, the lung tissues become more elastic and the muscles and joints of the ribs and spine become more supple.

Second, yoga asans stretch the thoracic cavity and strengthen postural muscles, contributing to

*See Funderburk, *Science Studies Yoga*, in Bibliography for reports of scientific studies of yoga.

an *increase in tidal volume*—the amount of air that flows in and out of the lungs in a normal resting state. As you read this, sit up straight and notice your breathing in its usual pattern. Now slouch down and see if you can notice how tidal volume is affected by poor posture.

A third way that yoga practice ensures that the body and brain receives enough oxygen is through *blood circulation*, one of the effects of yoga asans. The stretching of muscles that is accomplished through yoga also means increased elasticity of the blood vessels, allowing improved blood flow—and thus more oxygen—to all parts of the body.

How to Start Breathing Better

Posture. If there is one essential element to proper breathing, it is correct posture. Whether you sit cross-legged on the floor, or sit on your feet, or sit on the edge of a chair, it is important to keep your back straight but relaxed, so that you don't ache and start slouching after a few minutes (A). If your hips and knees are limber enough to allow you to sit cross-legged on the floor, be sure to sit on one or more firm pillows in order to allow your hips to tilt forward, making a slight arch in your lower back (B). You may use any of the illustrated cross-legged positions (CDEFG) that is comfortable. *Do not try to force your legs into a painful position before they are ready*; instead, do the hip- and

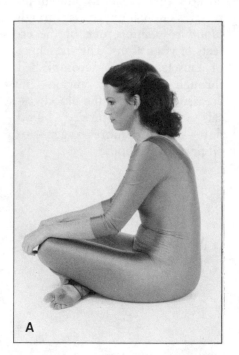

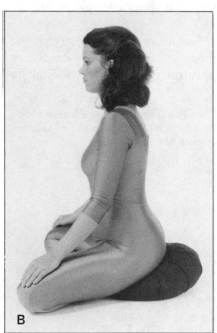

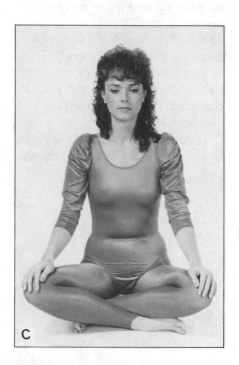

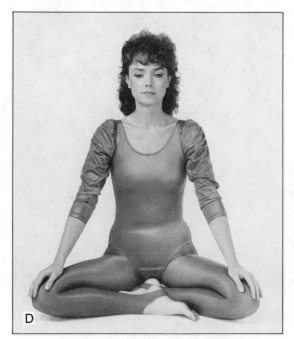

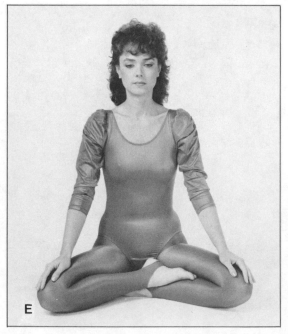

knee-limbering asans every day in your routine until all the joints in your legs loosen up.

If you are sitting in a chair, sit on the edge—do not lean back. Tuck your toes under so your thighs are inclined slightly (H); if your feet don't reach the floor, put a pillow or book under them. If you are sitting on your feet, a small pillow under your ankles and another under your hips will be more comfortable (I). You can also straddle a firm pillow so that your legs are bent slightly out to the sides (J).

Try each of the seated positions just described and see which feels more comfortable. Spend time on this now, and you will be rewarded by easier and quicker progress in your breathing.

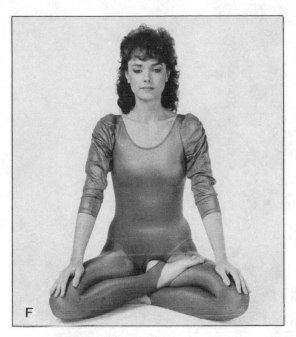

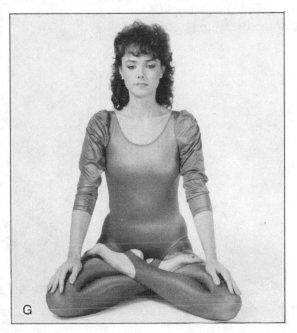

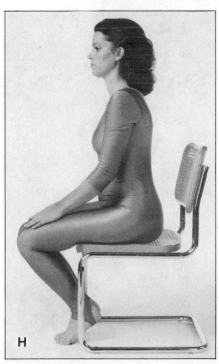

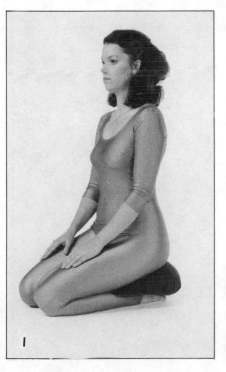

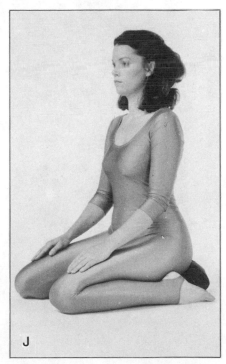

BREATH WARM-UPS

Always do these warm-ups before doing your breathing exercises: they will help loosen tight breathing muscles, relax your spine and get your circulation going. If your feet or legs get cramped after doing these exercises, stop and move around; massage your feet and ankles, and then sit again for the rest of the breathing exercises.

BACK ARCH

Slouch down so that your back is rounded as far forward as it will go, leaving your head face forward and hands resting on your knees. Breathe out (A). Now breathe in and arch your back forward, pushing your stomach out and jutting your chin out (B). Keep lips and teeth together. Then breathe out and slouch, remembering to keep your face forward; continue for several repetitions.

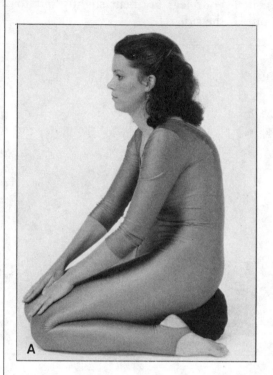

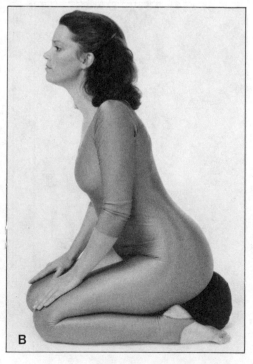

ARM SWING

Slouch forward as in the back arch, keeping your arms together in front of you, parallel to the floor. Breathe out, face forward (A). Now breathe in and push your stomach and back forward into an arch while swinging your arms out to the sides and as far back as they will go, keeping them straight and still parallel to the floor (B). Breathe out and slouch, bringing your hands together in front. Repeat several times. Variation: Bend elbows and bring arms back to the sides as if pulling back on the reins of a horse (C).

ARM REACH

Breathe out with arms at your sides (A). Now breathe in and bring your arms out to the sides and up over your head in a circular motion. Stretch your arms up as high as possible toward the ceiling (B). Breathe out and lower your arms to the sides again with the same circular motion. Repeat several times.

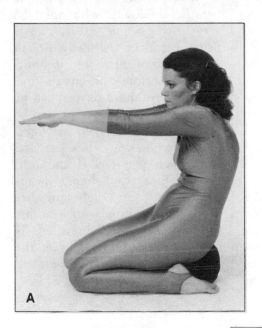

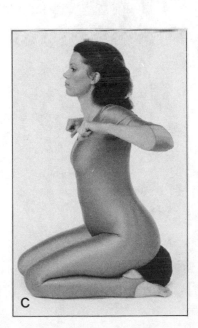

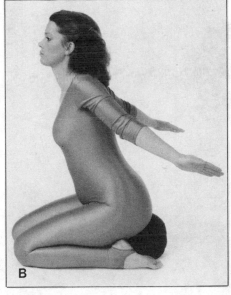

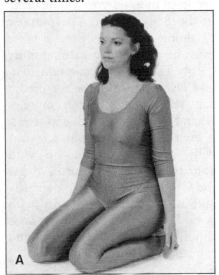

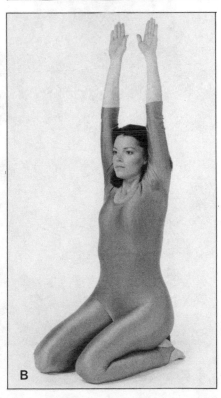

BREATHING EXERCISES

(Pranayamas)

BELLY BREATH

In a comfortable seated position, place both hands on your abdomen, just below your navel. Contract your abdominal muscles, then relax them. This is the main group of muscles you will be using in the Belly Breath. The purpose of doing the Belly Breath is to learn how to start breathing more deeply using the diaphragm first, and also to learn how the breath can relax the stomach muscles when they are tensed due to stress.

First exhale and contract your belly muscles, pushing in with your hands to help your body get the idea (A). Now relax your belly and inhale, pushing forward with your belly muscles—your hands should be pushed forward, and there should be a slight arch in your lower back (B). Now exhale again, push in with your hands and flatten your back (do not slouch on the exhalation; just come back to a straight-back position). Repeat several times, trying to inhale and exhale as completely as possible each time. Be sure to get some movement of your pelvis in this exercise by tilting forward so as to make a slight arch in the small of your back as you breathe in. Then return to a straight back as you tighten your stomach muscles and breathe out.

Do not hold your breath at any time, but make the breathing pattern smooth and steady. Breathe through your nose; you should feel the breath hitting the back of your throat first and hear a steamlike sound as the breath goes in and out. This sound is important, because achieving the proper sound helps you build up greater control of the breath using your throat muscles.

In this exercise you will experience your diaphragm moving first *down* to draw the air in and then *up* to expel the air. Most people breathe shallowly, with only the very top portion of the lungs being used. In the Belly Breath you are drawing more air down into the bottom portions of your lungs, where more oxygen can be absorbed into the bloodstream.

If you find that you get lightheaded while doing this exercise, stop when you feel it and rest. Feeling that way simply means that there is a slight pressure change going on in your head because of the increased oxygen. As you continue daily practice, the lightheadedness will disappear.

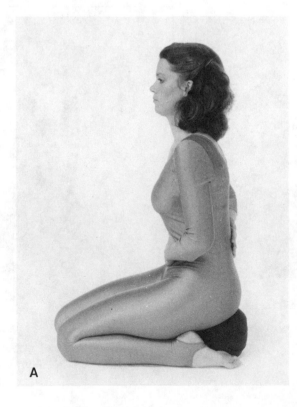

A

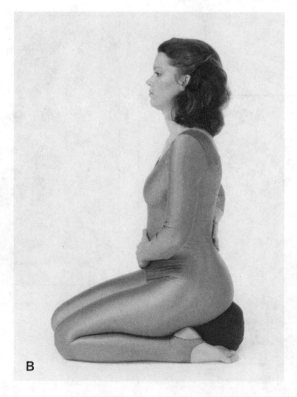

B

COMPLETE BREATH

This is the technique you will probably use most often to combat the tensions of stress in your life. The Complete Breath is a tool you can use anywhere, anytime, to calm your mind and relax from physical tension. Using the Complete Breath to center yourself before your meditation and even before your asans will make those aspects of practice even more effective.

The Complete Breath has three major parts. You have already learned the first, by doing the Belly Breath. The second is a bit more complicated. Place your hands on the lower part of your rib cage, with fingers just touching. The idea here is that as you breathe in, your rib cage will expand—not just forward but also *to the side*. When you achieve this you will notice a tremendous increase in your breath capacity. As you start to inhale, remember to push the belly forward and have a slight arch in the lower back. Continue to breathe in and try to expand your ribs sideways (A); your fingers should naturally come apart. Do not strain. Exhale (B), and your fingers should come together again. Breathe steadily for several repetitions, keeping your hands on your ribs. If you are breathing correctly, your fingers will be naturally and easily pulled apart a little as the ribs expand.

The third part of the Complete Breath concerns the top portion of the lungs. As you come to the top of your inhalation, straighten your shoulders and stretch your spine a little, and feel the breath being pushed into the very top of your lungs. Again, do not push too hard or you will strain the diaphragm and other muscles.

Put the three stages together for the Complete Breath inhalation (C) and reverse for exhalation (D). Inhalation is done from the bot-

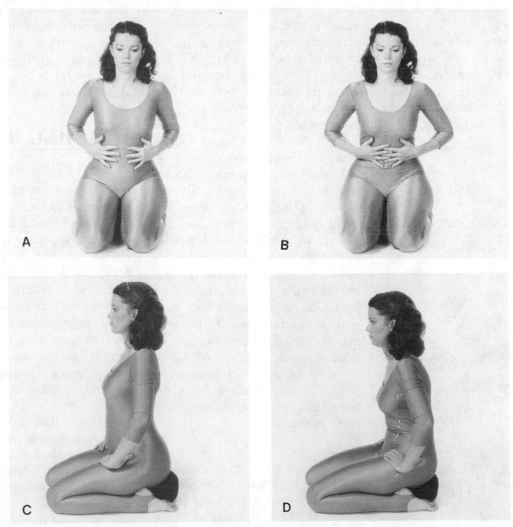

tom up and exhalation from the top down. Remember to breathe through your nose, concentrating on that steamlike sound in the back of your throat. Breathe evenly, without counting, and do not hold the breath at top or bottom. An important point about posture is that your shoulders and head should stay essentially in the same position throughout; try not to slouch forward on the exhalation, because then you will be using your spine as a bellows to expel the air instead of your muscles. Use the Wall Breath (E) to check your posture from time to time. Place a chair sideways against a wall and sit on it with your back against the wall. Be sure that your hips, shoulder blades and back of head are touching the wall. Start the Complete Breath with an exhalation, flattening the small of your back against the wall and tightening your stomach muscles. Now inhale and slightly arch your back as you fill up with air, using the

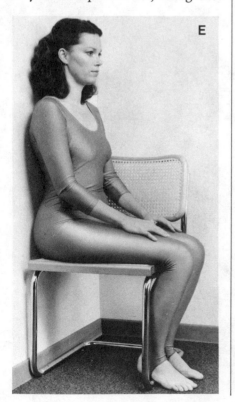

E

three stages. Your shoulders and head should remain against the wall at all times. Repeat several times.

After a couple of weeks start timing your breath, using a clock's second hand or a digital second readout. (If you don't have either of these, you may count silently in order to establish a proper rhythm.) Your inhalation and exhalation should be *about equal* in length in the Complete Breath, but be sure that you do not sacrifice correct form for length of time.

In the first ten weeks of curriculum, try for an even, comfortable 10 seconds of inhalation and 10 seconds of exhalation. You will probably notice that your inhalation is shorter than your exhalation. If that is the case, don't strain to extend the inhalation; instead, shorten your exhalation. Be sure not to hold your breath either at the top or the bottom, but make the transition smooth. Concentrate on the movement of your body and the sound of your breath. Evenness is more important than timing.

Practice the Complete Breath just before your meditation, to start the process of relaxation and begin to internalize your thoughts. Practicing this exercise lying on your back will also make it a bit easier to experience the proper movement of your stomach and back. As you breathe in, push your stomach up toward the ceiling. As you breathe out, tighten your stomach muscles and flatten the small of your back against the floor. Try this with a book on your stomach to strengthen your muscles even more.

EAR PLUGS

After you have practiced the Complete Breath for a few weeks, try it using earplugs. Your pharmacy probably has ear stopples

made of wax, beeswax or paraffin which are advertised on the box to reduce environmental noise. (You should *not* get the rubber earplugs used for swimming, which are less effective.) Yogis have traditionally used earplugs to help them achieve greater smoothness and control over their breath.

Try closing your ears with your fingers, and breathe deeply. Do you notice how much louder the breath sounds, overriding any distracting sounds? This is the purpose of using earplugs. To use them, knead them lightly to soften them, then flatten them on the outside of your ear canal. Don't push all the way in! Now practice your Complete Breath, trying to improve the evenness and smoothness of your breath.

You will probably find that this technique increases your concentration as well. If you wish, leave the earplugs in for meditation to reduce distracting noises.

HUMMING BREATH

The Humming Breath departs from the pattern of breathing you have done so far, in which the inhalation and exhalation are of approximately equal length. In the Humming Breath you will be breathing in for a short length of time and breathing out longer— as long as you can—while humming loudly and steadily. This exercise may seem strange at first, but it is extremely helpful in strengthening the diaphragm muscle and in quieting the mind for meditation.

Sitting comfortably, take in a full, quick Complete Breath (a little quicker than you usually do— about 3 to 5 seconds), but with the same movements of belly and chest. Now sing the word *hum* on one note and hold the *m* sound as you continue to exhale. Try to keep the tone steady and resonant until all your breath is gone. Then take in another deep, complete breath and start again. Repetitions: at least 5.

Choose a pitch that is comfortable for your voice. In the beginning you may notice that the note wavers quite a bit; that is because you are learning to control the "push" of your diaphragm all the way through the exhalation. Try not to let the sound die down at the end. You will have to push a little harder to keep a steady, resonant tone until the air has been completely exhaled.

BREATHING AND MOOD CHANGES

Earlier in this chapter we talked about the ability of breathing exercises to change mood. Some exercises are especially useful for this purpose.

One of the problems with "bad moods," whether depression, upset, anger or sadness, is that they act like a broken record in the body and mind, creating a vicious cycle of tense muscles, unproductive and negative thoughts, and constricted breathing. The following techniques are guaranteed to break that cycle and allow a more positive outlook to emerge.

THE LION

Sit on your feet (or the edge of a chair) with your hands on your knees (A). Take in a deep complete breath, then exhale with a growl, opening your eyes, mouth and hands wide, sticking out your tongue and leaning forward (B). Repeat several times!

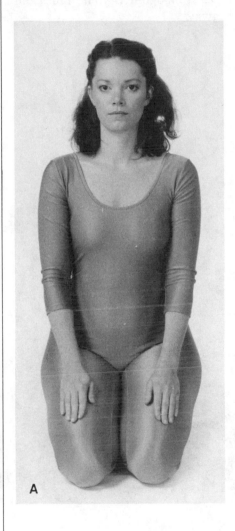

A

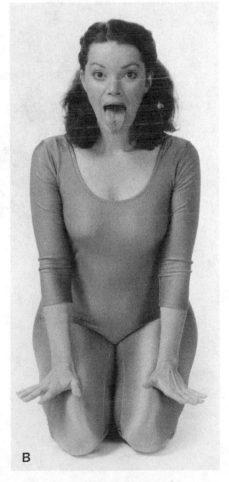

B

LAUGHASAN

This exercise can be done sitting in a chair, but it is most effective when you can move your whole body, as you can while lying down. Start your legs pumping as if you were riding a bicycle, pump your arms, make fists and laugh! Get your whole body involved. Even if you have to start by *pretending* to laugh, you will end up *really* laughing, your blues far away.

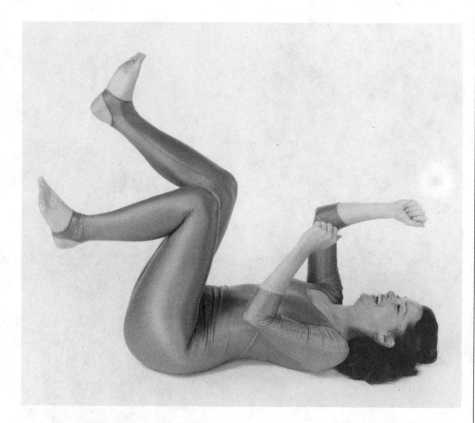

BREATHING EXERCISES NEW TO COURSE TWO

Neti

This is a cleansing technique for the sinus passages. It helps clear those areas so that breathing is facilitated, and it can also be helpful in shrinking swollen membranes. Are you aware of the fact that modern medicine recommends lots of sweet or salty liquids when you have a cold and sore throat? The reason is that these types of liquid have what is called osmotic action, meaning that they draw liquid out of mucous membranes and help shrink swelling, thereby easing discomfort. Neti acts in much the same way. Note: If you have allergies or a chronic sinus condition, do this technique only when the membranes are not inflamed.

You will need a styrofoam or paper cup and table salt. Put about a half-teaspoon of salt in the cup and fill about halfway with warm (*not cold*) water. Stir.

Now press the sides of the cup together slightly so that you create a spout. Holding one nostril closed with your other hand, tip the cup up toward your nose with your head slightly lifted. Inhale and tip the cup at the same time, sucking up a small amount of salt-water into your nose. Tilt your

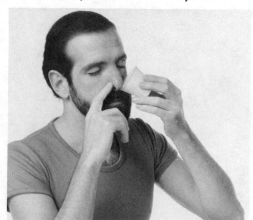

head back so the water runs through your sinuses. Soon you will feel it tickle the back of your throat. Don't swallow! Instead, lean over the sink and spit out the water. Repetitions: 1 to 3 times each side. Gently wipe your nose but don't blow hard for about five minutes.

It is not possible to drown from this technique! Practice it on a daily basis for a while and see if it makes your breathing more effective.

KAPALABHATI

This is an important breath technique because it helps prepare the mind for meditation. Literally, the word *kapalabhati* means "shining skull." Its other effects are to improve the nervous system coordination of the breath musculature, to relieve stress by releasing muscle tension in the chest and belly muscles, and to strengthen the diaphragm. Do not practice this technique when ill, during menstruation or if you are taking tranquilizers.

It is *mandatory* that your back be straight and your pelvis tilted forward so there is a slight arch in the small of your back. Your hips must be *higher* than your knees. This is important because you won't be able to get the proper movement if you are using your lower back or stomach muscles to maintain a comfortable seat.

Here is the beginning sequence, followed by an explanation of each item:
one-half normal breath inhalation, then:

1. 10 seconds bellows breath (approximately 1 per second)
2. complete, quick exhalation (3 to 5 seconds)
3. complete, quick inhalation (3 to 5 seconds)
4. hold breath in for 2 seconds
5. exhale as long as possible
6. 5 or more regular breaths, until breath is back to normal

1. Bellows Breath:

As its name implies, this action is a rapid in-and-out movement of the diaphragm. Place your hands just under your ribs in the center of your torso and breathe in and out a few times. This movement should not be the complete, belly-first type of breathing that you learned for the Complete Breath, but just an exercise in moving the diaphragm. You should feel the diaphragm expand as you breathe in and contract as you breathe out. For the Bellows Breath, start by breathing in to about one-half capacity and begin the bellows by exhaling. Take much smaller breaths than normal, but move enough air so that you get a definite sound. Remember that you should be using your diaphragm and *not* your belly for this exercise. Using your belly will make the bellows too forceful, possibly resulting in injury.

Notes on the sound: For previous breathing exercises we have been telling you to breathe making a sound in the back of your throat, by opening the throat muscles slightly. For the Bellows Breath you will need to make the sound from the tips of your nostrils instead. Relax your throat muscles to make this sound correctly. If you look in a mirror, you will notice your nostrils flaring slightly each time if you are doing the bellows correctly.

Notes on speed and intensity: For the first week concentrate on *evenness* in speed and intensity in this breath. Do not emphasize either the inhalation or the exhalation. The best way to ensure this is to start slowly: one in-out cycle each second for ten seconds. Try to make it a concentrated but very controlled burst of air both in and out, so that you are inhaling and exhaling the same *amount* of air. After a few weeks, if you are maintaining a smooth, even and steady bellows, increase the speed to two in-out breaths per second. After several weeks you can try increasing to three per second, but do not go faster than that.

Do you notice any lightheadedness after doing the bellows? If so, you may be using the top part of your chest rather than your diaphragm. Check by placing your hands on your chest. If you feel very much movement, try to relocate it to your diaphragm, just at the bottom of your rib cage. Heavy smokers may experience dizziness even if they are breathing correctly; if so, reduce the number of bellows you do at one time to five—or even fewer.

2. Quick Exhalation:

Use the same complete exhalation procedure as for the Complete Breath, only faster (3 to 5 seconds). Don't slouch. Use your stomach muscles. Get all the air out. From now on switch the *sound* of your breath to the back of your throat, making the steam-like sound you learned for the Complete Breath. The frontal nostril breath sound is for the bellows only.

3. Quick Inhalation:

Use the same inhalation procedure as in the Complete Breath, only faster (3 to 5 seconds). Fill from the bottom. Fill completely. Check your posture.

4. Hold Breath

This short (2 to 3 seconds) hold is to center or focus your awareness fully on the moment of stillness that is the transition between the inhalation and the exhalation.

5. Exhale As Long As Possible:

With this segment of the breath you enter the most absorbing and focused part of this exercise. The idea is to extend your exhalation as long as possible without strain. Imagine the breath coming out in the thinnest, softest stream you can imagine. Close your eyes to increase your concentration. Try to focus only on the sound of your breath (back of the throat). Be sure not to strain to the point of "squeaking" as you exhale. Also, don't extend the breath so much that you are starved for breath when finished. Stretch your exhalation a few seconds further each week. In the beginning, your exhalation will be fifteen to twenty seconds. By the time you have completed the Course Two ten-week session, if you've practiced

regularly, your exhalation will probably have grown to at least thirty seconds.

6. 5 or More Regular Breaths:

Release your breath and let it come naturally until the rate is back to normal and your muscles have relaxed (five or more breaths).

Repetitions:

Repeat the whole sequence three times to begin. If that feels comfortable, and you have extra time, you can increase to five repetitions after a few weeks.

Suggested Kapalabhati rate sequence during Course Two:

weeks 1 and 2: Bellows 10 seconds; whole sequence 3 times

weeks 3 and 4: Bellows 20 seconds; whole sequence 3 times

weeks 5 and 6: Bellows 20 seconds but increase speed to 2 per second; whole sequence 3 times

weeks 7 and 8: Bellows 30 seconds; whole sequence 5 times

weeks 9 and 10: Bellows 30 seconds; increase speed to 3 per second if ready; whole sequence 5 times

---

BRAMARI BREATH

This is a focusing exercise that demands attention, much like the Humming Breath, because you have to make an audible sound. In this case it is an extended "zzz" sound, hence its name, which means "bee breath."

Start by placing your fingers as in the illustration: thumbs on the flap in front of the ear; first finger on the eyelashes of your closed eyes; second finger at the nostrils; third and fourth fingers at the corners of the mouth. Fingers should be placed lightly, not pressed hard. By symbolically closing your sensory input organs, you will reinforce the idea of focusing on the sound of the breath alone. Do *not* apply pressure, except with your thumbs, which should *gently* close the ear openings on the exhalation so that the sound is intensified.

Inhale completely through your nose, using all three steps as in the Complete Breath. As you exhale, press your thumbs softly to close the ears and make the "zzz"

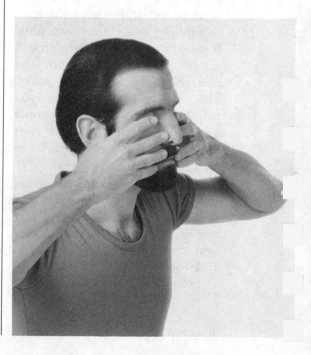

sound, extending the breath and keeping the tone steady until you run out of air. Repetitions: 3 to 5.

Most students find this to be an excellent technique for changing moods, because it forces concentration away from the bad mood —sort of like nudging the needle that is stuck on a broken record —and clears the mind to go on to more constructive and positive things. In addition, the exercise helps quiet the mind for meditation because of its focusing effects.

BREATHING EXERCISES NEW TO COURSE THREE

SPINAL ARCH

The Spinal Arch stimulates the nerves of the entire spinal column and places pressure on the rib cage and lungs, allowing more oxygen to be absorbed through the lung walls. It is part of the Emotional Stability Routine (Course Three).

Sit cross-legged, and place your fists on the floor directly behind your hips (A). Take a partial breath in (to about one-half normal capacity), straighten your arms so that you are lifting a little of your weight off your buttocks, arch your back slightly, tuck your chin to your chest and contract your rectal muscles (B). This contraction is called the *mulabhanda* lock. Hold your breath and the pose for three to six seconds. Release and relax. Repetitions: 3

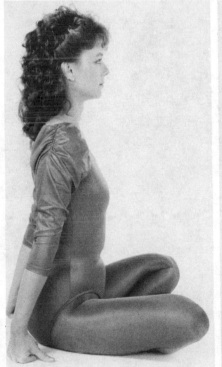

A

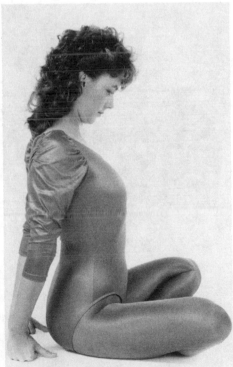

B

AGNI KRIYA

This is an advanced breath exercise that should only be attempted after you have become proficient in Kapalabhati. Agni Kriya involves what is called a *bandha*, or "lock," of a part of the body, in order to intensify a movement or limitation of movement of energy. In Agni Kriya you have to practice isolating stomach and diaphragm muscles. This is a powerful technique that should never be done on a full stomach, by pregnant women or by menstruating women.

First practice this exercise from a standing position. Place your hands on your bent knees, as in the illustration (A), bracing yourself but relaxed. Breathe in deeply, filling your lungs as full as possible; then breathe out very quickly, through pursed lips. Did you get all the air out? Try to exhale a little more. Now hold your breath out and pull in and up with your stomach muscles, contracting them so that the triangular area under your rib cage becomes slightly hollow (B). Hold for a moment. Now release your muscles and lift your chin a little. When your muscles are completely relaxed, *then* release your held breath and breathe in. Relax until your breath returns to normal (take five or more normal, resting breaths).

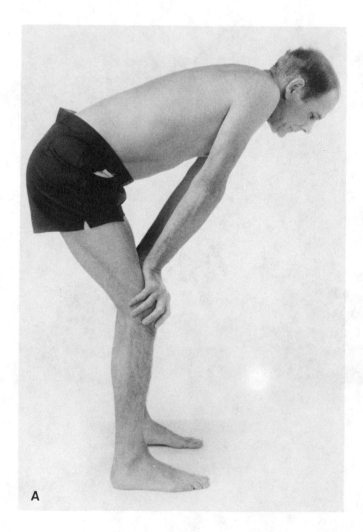

A

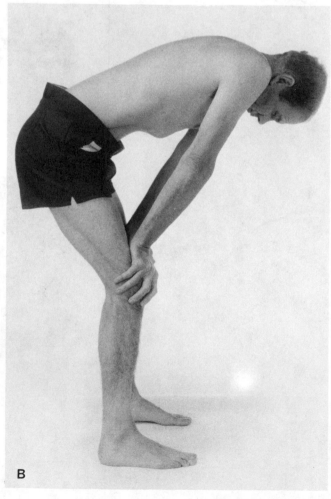

B

Practice three repetitions of this first step after your other breath exercises every day. If you experience headaches, nervousness, pain in the diaphragm or dizziness, stop the exercise; your nervous system is not yet strong enough to support it. Continue with daily asans, Complete Breath and Kapalabhati, and try again in a few weeks.

If you experience none of these symptoms after a week, begin repetitions of the stomach contraction as follows: Exhale completely through pursed lips, hold the breath out, draw the stomach up and in, hold for a moment, then release the stomach muscles but *not* the held breath. Contract the stomach again; release; contract a third time; release. Relax the stomach muscles completely, then breathe in and relax until breath returns to normal (five or more normal, resting breaths). This is one repetition. Repetitions: 3.

After practicing the exercise standing for a while, try it seated (C & D). Make sure that your hips are higher than your knees, so use a pillow or two or sit on your feet, as in the illustration. You can also do this seated on the edge of a sturdy chair.

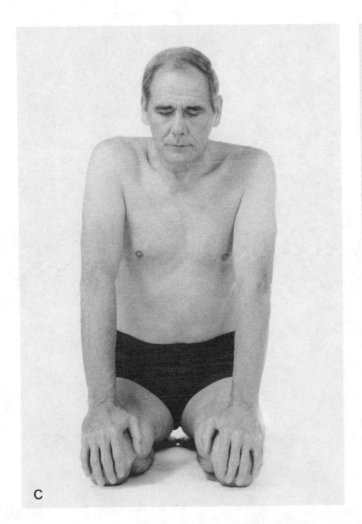

C

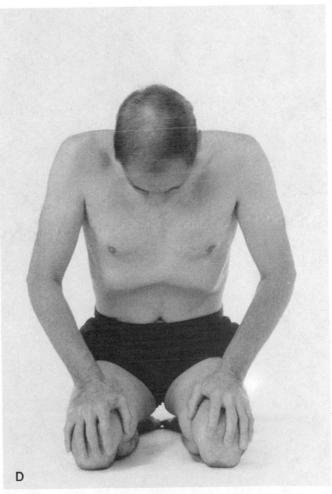

D

CHAPTER 6
RELAXATION AND MEDITATION

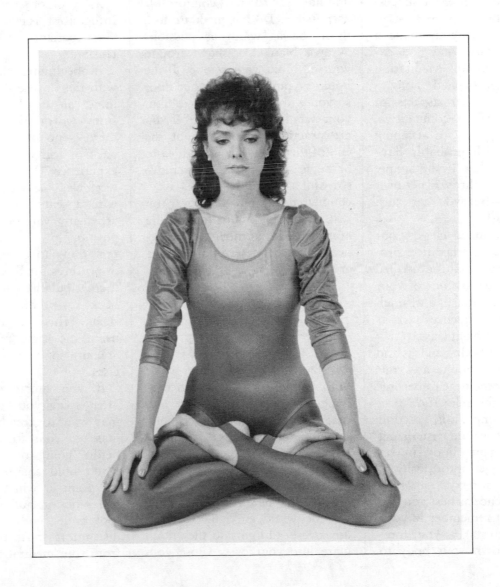

MEDITATION

Meditation is very difficult to teach because it is the one technique a teacher cannot *show* you. And because each person's experience will be slightly different, it is important for you to try not to be too judgmental about comparing your experiences to others'. The important thing to remember is that meditation progress is cumulative; even if you *think* that nothing is happening, the daily effort is increasing your concentration and willpower and getting your mind used to the idea of being still. "Play" with your meditation practice; try the different suggestions that follow for helping to make it work for you; make a game out of observing and exploring your mind. Meditation should be approached nonviolently, just as other aspects of yoga. If you take a competitive, forceful attitude toward attaining stillness, you will probably have more difficulty than if you simply let go. You can't throw a net over a whirlwind—but you can turn your back on it!

If you are in a class, your teacher will use a relaxation procedure similar to what is described here. To get the most out of your daily practice sessions, go through the relaxation sequence just as you remember it from class.

If you are not taking a class and are using this book as your teacher, take some time to become familiar with the relaxation process by reading this section through carefully and visualizing each part of your body in sequence. Then get into position, close your eyes and try to approximate the sequence as best you can remember. Just remember in your visualizations to start at your forehead, move down your body to your toes and then come back up your spine to your head. Don't worry if you forget one or two points, but be sure to spend adequate time on relaxation (at least four minutes) before moving on to your meditation.

Alternatively, you may wish to read the instructions slowly into a tape recorder to play back while you relax. A prerecorded tape is available from the American Yoga Association.

It is important to take the time to relax completely, because that starts the process of internalization. Use your yoga mat or blanket, wear your exercise clothes and have the room as comfortable as possible. Do not meditate in a draft; be as warm as possible. Wrap a blanket or shawl around yourself. Take your phone off the hook, or put a sign on your door so you will not be disturbed. Shut your pets in another room. If you are practicing meditation at the end of the day, it is a good idea to bathe first, to relax and remove stressful associations that have accumulated during the day. You will find other hints for getting more out of your meditation practice after the description of the process itself.

HOW TO BEGIN

1. Get into Position

Start your meditation practice by lying down on your back on your mat or blanket. (See the chapter on stress for a shorter seated meditation procedure that you can use at any time of day.) If your blanket is shorter than you are, your head should be on it. Be sure you will be warm enough. Turn off any overhead lights so they don't glare into your eyes. Close your eyes. Do not use a pillow unless, because of injury or your doctor's orders, you must keep your head elevated. Let your arms relax at your sides, with the palms of your hands facing up. Let your legs and feet relax. Check to make sure that your body is very straight. This position is called the Corpse Pose (Shavasan) because the body gets so completely relaxed that it is almost motionless—only a slight breathing motion is apparent.

If you wish, you may vary this position by bending your knees and placing your feet about a foot apart, so that your knees touch. This position, called the Easy Bridge Rest, is especially helpful if you experience lower back pain or tension.

In beginning classes we start with the Corpse Pose because the mind can then be completely free from worry about the body—there is no discomfort from the back or legs to intrude upon the experience. In the second ten-week class we begin to experiment with a seated meditation. There are many variations to a seated position (p. 132), but the important thing to remember—just as in postures for breathing—is that there should be a slight arch in the back to prevent slouching and strain. This can be ensured by using the same pillow structure you use for your breathing exercises.

If you meditate immediately after doing your breathing, you may want to stretch your legs and massage your knees and ankles before going on to meditation. Don't hold a sitting position to the point at which you begin to feel pain or numbness, or your foot or leg goes to sleep! When discomfort starts to distract you from your meditation, gently shift to the Corpse Pose or Easy Bridge Rest without opening your eyes and with as little movement as possible. Then quickly go through the relaxation process that follows, checking to make sure that the special tension trouble areas such as the breath, face and stomach are relaxed, and continue your meditation.

2. Relax Completely

Spend 4 to 6 minutes on this process, going through the steps in the following outline. Don't skip this section; unless your body is relaxed and still, it will be much harder to quiet your mind. Don't worry if you cannot recall the entire procedure; just remember to move your attention slowly from your forehead down to your toes, and back up your spine to your head, relaxing each part individually.

First, mentally detach yourself from all the activities, responsibilities and cares that occupy you during the day. Say to yourself, "For a few minutes I don't have to speak, move or respond to anyone or anything. I don't even have to think. I can become completely still and relaxed."

FACE

To begin your relaxation, bring your concentration or attention to the area of your forehead between the eyebrows and quietly imagine a diamondlike dot of light. This is the part of the body that represents a stage of consciousness called the *ajna chakra*, a state in which intuitive wisdom comes forward and can be more easily used. If you can't imagine this light, or if it makes you uncomfortable, just concentrate your attention on that area between your eyebrows.

Now take your attention down your nose bone and across your eyebrows, relaxing them. Let the force of gravity and your attention relax all the muscles in the forehead and eyes. The eyes merit special attention because they are the center for perception, the primary sense organ through which we perceive and respond to the world. Once your eyes are relaxed, try not to allow them to move back and forth under your lids until you want them to. Allow your eyes to sink back into the eye sockets until the muscles and nerves feel completely stilled. This may take some practice but it can and will be accomplished successfully.

Move your attention across your cheeks, relaxing the muscles underneath your skin. Focus for a few seconds on the hinge of your jaw, located just in front of your ear. Relax your jaw as much as possible. You can even let your mouth hang open slightly to relax your lower jaw as much as possible. Relax your mouth, picturing your teeth, tongue and throat, and remind yourself that you don't have to speak for a few minutes. Now move your attention to your neck and throat. Imagine that your face and throat are made out of warm, soft wax.

SHOULDERS, ARMS, HANDS

Next, move your attention across your collarbone, relaxing it, and to your shoulder joints. Pause for a moment and picture your shoulder joint loosening and relaxing. Direct your attention down your arms. Picture the long bones in your arms, the skin, muscles, nerves and veins in your elbows all becoming still and relaxed. Imagine your wrists and hands floating in water. Don't move your hands; just relax them from the inside with your mind. Visualize the position of your hands, the shape of your fingers and nails, the lines in your hands, and then let them go limp, as if they were a pair of empty gloves lying next to you on the floor.

HEART AND LUNGS

Gently redirect your attention to your chest. Picture your heart pumping steadily, day in and day out; then take a deep breath, and as you exhale, imagine your heart relaxing even more than it already has. It doesn't have to beat quite as hard now for a few minutes.

BREATH

Observe how your breathing pattern is becoming more and more relaxed. Take another deep breath. As you fill your lungs, picture them as bright, strong and healthy, and exhale in a long sigh, letting your lungs relax back into your natural breath pattern. Don't try to slow or speed up your breath; let your breath become smooth, quiet and rhythmic, free of all tension or strain.

STOMACH AND INTERNAL ORGANS

Even if you aren't quite sure what they look like, picture your internal organs—your stomach, liver, kidneys, intestines, etc., and relax them also. Imagine them working perfectly. Let your insides gently sink toward your backbone.

HIPS, LEGS, FEET

Let the bones, muscles, glands and nerves of your hips and hip joints all become still and free of strain or tension. Continue down your legs, picturing the long muscles, nerves and bones sinking limply toward the floor, like warm putty. Relax the joints of the knees, picturing the veins. Relax your ankles, feet and toes, and picture your toes. Think of their shape and the position of your feet. Let your feet become limp and relaxed. Relax your heels where they touch the floor, and even relax the floor; you should feel a relaxed *environment* as well as body.

SPINAL COLUMN

Gently bring your attention to and relax the base of your spine. Picture your spinal column as a gently curving elevator with the spinal cord running up inside it like a shiny cord of electricity up to the brain. Relax your spinal column nerves and bones from your lower back up to the back of your neck. Then relax the spot where your spinal column joins your skull. Release the back of your neck from any tension. Picture the brain and let it become absolutely relaxed. Feel as though it is relaxing and settling quietly into your skull.

RECHECK FACE

Check your face for any lingering tension, especially in the area of your eyes. Make sure your jaw is relaxed. Now gently bring your attention back to the space in the forehead between the eyebrows. Your whole body is now quiet and relaxed.

3. Think of the Sound *Om*

Om (pronounced "ohm") is a *mantram*. A mantram is a very particular sound—a form of energy, in fact—that focuses the mind and is used to elicit a specific result. *Om* is a mantram that has been used as an aid to meditation during the thousands of years of yoga's history because it centers and focuses the mind on the silence of meditation. A teacher may use the sound *om* at the beginning and end of meditation to facilitate the transition. In your meditation practice at home, try repeating the sound mentally a few times after you complete your relaxation. You should find that it helps you become quieter easier and more quickly.

4. Be quiet and still for 10 to 20 minutes

As your attention begins to shift from your relaxed body to your mind, begin to observe and detach yourself from involvement with your thoughts. Meditation is a state of complete stillness and inactivity within the conscious mind. There may still be thoughts and perceptions moving at the edges of your awareness, but your attention is not on that movement but rather on the silence and stillness that surrounds and underlies the mind.

5. Helpful Hints

Meditation is not the same as being unconscious. In meditation, your body is completely relaxed, just as it is in sleep, but your mind is attentive, concentrated, alert and poised. Try to adopt an attitude of playfulness, instead of a forceful one of pushing or pressing against your thoughts. Remember that you are attempting to train your mind to be still—something that is, for most people, a completely new experience, unlike anything they have attempted before. Like any other type of training, meditation takes practice.

At first you will become aware of stillness "after the fact," when you start thinking and realize that you have *not* been thinking for a few seconds previously. If you catch yourself in the middle of a thought, finish it but then consciously let it fade away and try to focus on the space before the next thought intrudes. Try to experience the silence as a feeling, or even, if it is easier for you, imagine the characteristics of the silence—its wideness, deepness, thickness, texture, and so on.

Even if you feel that you are still only for a few seconds at a time at first, those periods of time will gradually lengthen and widen, and the experience of stillness will be engrossing and pleasant.

Sometimes, at first, you may fall asleep. If this happens to you, just remember that as you begin to meditate, you are giving your body all the cues that it associates with sleep—a darkened room, relaxing the body, lying down, eyes closed—so it is natural for you to slip into this state sometimes, especially if you are very fatigued. If this happens to you, you will probably notice that it is a different kind of sleep than usual—probably deeper and more restful, and usually without dreams. You will also notice (unless you are extremely tired) that you will tend to wake up spontaneously after twenty or thirty minutes feeling refreshed.

Try not to set an alarm when you meditate, because the loud sound will jar your nervous system and startle you awake too violently. If you meditate in the morning and are afraid you will fall asleep and be late, there are a few ways to help. First, you may wish to consider sitting up for your meditation. (See p. 132 for seated positions.) Second, set an alarm for about ten minutes *after* you usually end your meditation, and put the alarm under a pillow or in a drawer so the sound is somewhat muffled. Chances are, you will wake up after your usual time is over, but the alarm provides a safeguard.

Sometimes there may be so many thoughts going through your mind that you find it impossible to detach yourself from them. There will be days in everyone's life when so much is going on that it is very hard to be still. On those days you may wish to try using an image of some kind to help relax and quiet your mind. To do this, pick an image that gives you a quiet feeling, such as a lake, ocean, meadow, sky, or the like, and visualize that image until you experience the same kind of quiet feeling. Then gently let go of the image—just let it dissolve—and let the quiet feeling remain as long as you can. Go back to your image as often as you need to in order to remain still. Be careful, however, that you don't get so involved in the image that your mind gets carried away by memories and perceptions associated with that image!

In the chapter on breathing you read about using earplugs to increase your concentration on the sound of your breath. You can, if you wish, also use the earplugs for your meditation if you are bothered by noises outside your room.

One phenomenon related to this problem that is common to many students is that in the beginning stages of meditation practice, external sounds, such as a clock, traffic, an air conditioner or some such, suddenly become (or seem to become) much louder. This is because you are now quieting all the surface mental conversation that normally goes on all the time in your mind without you being aware of it. When you consciously subdue that mental activity, its screening effect disappears and you suddenly become much more aware of external sounds. After a while, however, you will learn to habituate to (tune out) those external sounds so they don't bother you anymore.

6. Coming Out of Meditation

When your meditation period is over, think again of the sound *om*. Then, before you move, try to remember how it felt to be still in-side. Remembrance of that feeling is the first step in being able to re-create it whenever you need or want it during the day.

Never jump right up after your meditation. Start by changing your breathing pattern. Breathe a little more deeply, and picture the air filling and "waking up" your body. Find your hands and wiggle your fingers. Make a fist. Find your feet, and wiggle your toes. Pull your toes back toward your face so you feel a stretch up the back of your legs. Whenever you are ready, slowly start to stretch and move about.

BENEFITS OF MEDITATION IN EVERYDAY LIFE

If you practice meditation every day, even for just a few minutes, you will soon notice that the rest and relaxation that you feel begin to suffuse your entire life. These periods of stillness can be as refreshing as an hour's nap, because for a few minutes you are taking a mental vacation from all the cares, responsibilities, upsets, concerns, conversations and involvements of your daily life. The practice of yoga enables you gradually to attain control over your own mind—over the thoughts, dialogues and emotional upsets that revolve incessantly in your mental conversation. This control is tremendously helpful in reducing such debilitating feelings as anger, fear, depression, negativity and boredom. Through yoga, you become a truly whole, integrated person, able to face the many stresses of life, well fortified with strength and balanced judgment.

In most people, emotional upsets are the subject of most of these internal conversations, which in turn feed and prolong the upset, sapping your energy as well. Meditation helps break this destructive cycle by giving you a mental vacation in which the mind simply rests. Then, when you return to your everyday concerns, you get a new look at your mind's reactions to them; this gives you a fresh, possibly more effective approach to your problems.

Yoga teaches that the mind assumes the shape of whatever thought occupies it, just as water takes on the shape of whatever container it is in. The mind changes its shape through perception, imagination, desire, emotion, daydream, reasoning and many other mental processes. These are like waves or ripples on the surface of a pond, distorting or obscuring the view of the bottom. Meditation is the quieting of those mental thought waves so that your perception is clear. In yoga, your view of yourself is only accurate when you can detach yourself momentarily from *all* activity—physical, mental, emotional. When you are able to do this, you experience a clear and powerful insight into your true self, undistorted by the turbulence of personality. With this insight comes an inner happiness. You no longer have to depend totally on other people, or on going places, buying things, eating and drinking, or taking drugs. Happiness comes from within you.

COMMON EXPERIENCES IN MEDITATION

PART OF YOUR BODY—OR ALL OF IT—SEEMS TO DISAPPEAR:

When you completely relax in meditation, you will be withdrawing all your senses—including the kinesthetic sense, which is the awareness of where your body is in space. In meditation, that body consciousness is not needed and is withdrawn.

YOU FEEL LIGHT OR HEAVY:
When your awareness begins to shift away from the physical into the mental, you sometimes experience that as a heaviness or a lightness. The experience is similar to the feeling of falling when going to sleep that sometimes jerks your body awake.

YOU SEE LIGHTS OR COLORS, OR HEAR SOUNDS
Seeing or hearing things in meditation is often a very seductive experience, because it is so different from ordinary experience. This type of experience is caused by becoming more aware of the electrical activity in the brain, which then manifests as light or sound. You may read about the meanings of different colors and images, but we encourage students simply to note—and possibly record—these experiences, treat them as thoughts and go on toward your exploration of stillness, no matter how interesting they are.

A SOLUTION TO A PROBLEM SUDDENLY OCCURS TO YOU
If you have ever had the experience of going to sleep with a problem unsolved and waking up with the answer, you will understand the similarity in meditation. When you relax completely, quieting your surface emotions that usually churn like the waves on a lake, you will find that parts of your mind that ordinarily lie unused often emerge with a new clarity. Intuition, creativity and many other qualities that most people possess but rarely know how to use can be released this way. Although you shouldn't think of your meditation as a problem-solving session, you might consider keeping a pad of paper and a pen close at hand so that if something important occurs to you, you can write it down and forget about it, and go on with your meditation in stillness, instead of ending your meditation early or being anxious about holding on to that solution so that you won't forget it.

YOU FEEL COLD OR HOT
Feeling cold is a response to a natural drop in body temperature, which happens when you relax as if you were going to sleep. This is why you should be careful to stay warm when you meditate. Feeling hot is often a result of involuntary stimulation of the parasympathetic nervous system, which controls circulation and temperature.

YOUR EYES KEEP TWITCHING
The eye muscles are many times the last muscle group in your body to relax, because they are an important center of perception. You may notice a correlation between periods of thought and movement of your eyes—similar to the rapid eye movement (REM) which occurs during dreams while you are asleep. As your ability to detach yourself from involvement with your thoughts improves, your eye muscles will gradually relax. If the difficulty persists, it may be wise to check your diet; a B vitamin deficiency may be indicated.

NOTE:
A cassette tape of the relaxation and meditation procedure led by Alice Christensen is available by writing to The American Yoga Association.

CHAPTER 7
YOGA AND NUTRITION

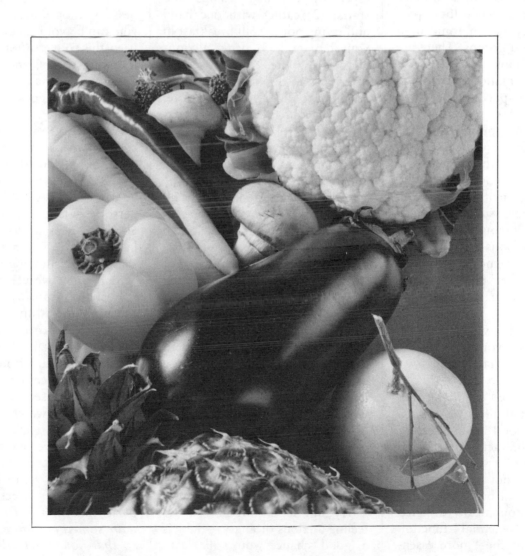

A YOGA PERSPECTIVE ON HEALTHY EATING

Practicing yoga seriously takes energy. Doesn't it just make sense to feed your body the foods that will reinforce your desire to improve your health, instead of working at cross-purposes? This chapter describes a commonsense approach to eating better.

THE YOGA DIET, OR IMPROVING YOUR NUTRITIONAL LIFE-STYLE

The yoga diet is not a miracle cure, a quick-weight-loss program, a fancy health tonic or a lecture on food groups. There are many other books that can give you more information of that kind than we have space for here (see Bibliography for sources). The yoga diet is an approach to eating from the point of view of a yogi that incorporates the principles of common sense, good health and stress management. It will also touch on subjects such as vegetarianism, food cravings, alternatives to traditional foods and the effects of food on your emotions.

The yoga diet takes into account first and foremost your *nutritional life-style*. This has to do with where and how you eat, your state of mind, your reasons for eating and only later with *what* you eat.

The importance of monitoring your nutritional life-style has to do with how food is absorbed by your body. The fact is, if you are in the middle of a stress reaction, your food will not be digested as well as it should be, because circulation is automatically diverted from the "less essential" function of digestion to the "more essential" areas of muscle tone and glandular function, in order to cope with the more immediate demand made by a stressor. (See the chapter on Yoga and Stress Management for specific responses the body makes during stress reactions.)

Remembering that a stressor can be emotional as well as physical, consider how many times during the day the body goes into a stress-reactive state. For example, if you eat breakfast in the car on the way to work, there are multiple stressors involved. These include (1) the extra attention you must give to driving in traffic, especially the many stops and starts; (2) eating with one hand and trying not to spill breakfast in your lap; and (3) being anxious about being late. Your body's first priority is to respond to the stressors, not to digest food; therefore, much of your breakfast may pass through your system partially undigested, causing unpleasant physical symptoms and robbing your system of valuable nutrients. The same goes for eating in a hurry, on your feet; in this case lateness anxiety causes your body to go through its usual stress responses, diverting circulation from your stomach, where digestion is going on, to the more vital functions.

So, no matter how nourishing your breakfast may be in theory, the amount of that nourishment that your body can actually use depends a lot on your state of mind, environment and motives while eating. For each eating occasion, *make your environment as pleasant as possible*. Set a place for yourself that is attractive and clean. If you don't have time to set a place, at least sit down to eat.

Try not to eat when you are feeling anxious or angry—there is a good chance you will "eat" those feelings, too, and intensify them! Because emotional anxieties cause physical stress reactions, they will naturally interfere with digestion as well. A good way to diffuse these feelings is to use water. Lightly wash your face and hands, mentally imagining the water to be rinsing off your anxieties. (See the chapter on stress for a fuller discussion of how to use water to affect how you feel.) Take a few deep breaths and mentally put all the troubles in another room. Resolve to enjoy your meal and not think about your problems while you eat.

Try not to discuss business while you eat, especially if business has a lot of tension for you. If you can't avoid it, at least try to keep the conversation away from upsetting topics, and you will be doing everyone a favor!

The same goes for cooking while you are feeling disturbed. Have you ever sat down to a meal cooked by someone who was angry about something? Somehow the food doesn't taste quite as good as that cooked by a happier person. When you cook, think about a pleasant topic, or, even better, think about a yoga concept that you are studying.

Sometimes we use food unconsciously to soothe and tranquilize; as circulation is diverted from the brain to the process of digestion, the edge is taken off our preoccupation with our trouble. If you find yourself eating more when you are depressed or bored, or as a habit while watching television or reading, you may be training your body to recognize food as a form of emotional support rather than simply nourishment. To counteract that effect, *try to replace your habitual eating habits with something more productive, so that you don't add unwanted pounds.*

Yoga's attitude toward food

echoes the concept of nonviolence, just as in other areas of life. *Your diet should not be a hardship*, nor should it take so much of your energy that you take time away from more important things. Decide which aspects of your diet you want to uphold rigorously and in which areas you will allow yourself a wider margin for deviation. (Read more about nonviolence later in this chapter, in the discussion about vegetarianism.)

Remember that as you start to change your diet for the better, a gradual changeover is more effective than changing all at once. Pick one new aspect each week to modify. Changing your diet all at once can be a powerful stressor in itself. Give your body and mind time to adjust to the new foods and eating patterns. Use your common sense.

Obviously, the *earlier you start on a new diet program, the better*. It would be nice if we could go back, with our new knowledge of what's good for us, and feed our bodies the right stuff from the beginning! But wherever you are in your life's journey, starting *right now* to change your diet will increase your chances of *not* having to change it radically when you are older. Even though diet is not the only determining factor in such conditions as high blood pressure, heart disease, digestive problems and so on, it is an important one. Starting now to reduce your intake of sodium and cholesterol, excess sugar, caffeine and alcohol, and to increase fiber sources, alternatives to meat proteins, widening your choices and adjusting to new caloric and nutrient levels will make a big difference later if you are required to adjust your diet more strictly as a result of some physical problem.

What starts as a discipline will gradually become habit. For example, if you slowly reduce the amount of sugar in your diet, you will enjoy the tastes of different foods more and won't crave sweets. Your sweet tooth will change also: While you may need two spoons of sugar for your tea to taste sweet now, later you may need only half a spoonful, and more will taste *too sweet*. You may even grow to enjoy tea with *no* added sweetener.

Breakfast

Breakfast is important! Would you start out on an automobile trip with an empty gas tank, thinking that you'd fill up when you reached your destination? Of course not. Yet so often we skip the first meal of the day because we "don't have time or energy." Yet for most people the important work gets done in the morning. We then find ourselves expecting our minds to function at top efficiency while running on last night's supply of fuel!

When the body is forced to draw on reserves of protein for energy, protein is taken first from the vital stress glands, the adrenals; then from the thymus and lymph glands; and finally from the muscles themselves. This causes a tremendous stress on the body, because the adrenals are supposed to be the center for fighting stress—not causing it themselves. So do your body a favor and "gas up" before you start work.

Having a good breakfast does not mean that it has to be a full production, taking time and effort that most people don't have in the morning. Start by compiling a list of menus for alternative breakfasts (suggestions follow) and keep the ingredients on hand at all times. This avoids eating junk just because it's convenient.

Breakfast should consist of proteins and "quality" carbohydrates—the carbohydrates that are more complex and break down more slowly into the bloodstream. They will produce energy both immediately and over several hours, so that you are fueled until lunchtime. Be creative; you're not limited to the "traditional" breakfasts of cereal, toast, eggs and orange juice. If you're a baker, try different breads and muffins—they freeze very well and heat up in minutes in a toaster oven or microwave oven. If you're not a baker, check the frozen foods or prepared foods section of your supermarket or specialty shop. Experiment with different fruit tastes: Try exotic varieties such as kiwi, pineapple and so on. Try making a blender drink with various fruits and juices. Make your own granola, to have with plain yogurt and possibly some fruit. (Making your own has a big advantage in that you can control the amount of sugar.) Even experiment with having leftover casseroles or other main dishes for breakfast. Who says breakfast has to be dull!

Since eating several smaller meals is much better than eating a few large ones during a day, a good alternative is to eat most of your breakfast at breakfast time, having the rest for your midmorning snack. That way you will avoid stuffing in unneeded calories with coffee and sweet snacks, which cause wild blood sugar swings and subject your body to even more stress.

Snacks

The right snacks—those that break down slowly—can extend your energy level. The wrong ones will give you a quick energy boost, as blood sugar skyrockets; then energy dives lower than before, as your body reacts by demanding insulin to remove the excess sugar, leaving you with low blood sugar symptoms. Learning wise snacking habits can make a big difference in the quality of your work and the state of your mind.

Recent research has changed the traditional ideas about which foods are better than others for controlling blood sugar.* Rather than relying on the old standards of "simple" versus "complex" carbohydrates, nutritionists are switching to a new standard based on the rate at which carbohydrates are broken down and absorbed into the bloodstream. It seems that some of the complex carbohydrates that have been recommended for dieters and diabetics, among others, are in fact, faster at releasing sugars into the bloodstream than are some of the simpler forms. For example, carrots and potatoes break down much faster than ice cream does! Ice cream, because it is mostly milk fat, breaks down much more slowly. So even though ice cream may be a less desirable food because of the fat and calorie content, it would be a better alternative than potatoes if you happen to be caught hungry in the shopping mall!

At work, keep some healthy snacks on hand, and discipline yourself to just *snack* rather than gulp down huge quantities of nuts or other goodies before your appetite control has registered "full." Snacks should be high-protein sources (protein may help

*Kolata, Gina, and Goldfarb, Toni, "In Praise of Pasta and Beans," *American Health*, Vol. II, No. 3, May/June, 1983.

you remain alert). Some fat content as well helps slow down the digestive process so you don't feel hungry so soon after eating.

Some examples of high-protein snacks: yogurt; low-fat cheese; dry roasted or low-salt (or no-salt) nuts, perhaps mixed with raisins, seeds, roasted soybeans and other goodies (but beware of eating too many dried fruits at one time—they have an extremely high sugar content, and many are processed with sulphites, to which some people are allergic); peanut butter. Most of these suggested snacks can be purchased in the supermarket. Finally, snacks should be low in salt, and you should be sure to drink plenty of liquids throughout the day.

If you normally have a snack in the evening (easily allowable if you count this as the sixth small meal of the day and have allocated calories appropriately), have a high-carbohydrate snack, such as whole-grain crackers and peanut butter, or an apple with a little cheese or granola with some yogurt. Carbohydrates increase the brain's absorption of the amino acid tryptophan, which stimulates production of serotonin. This neurotransmitter has a hypnotic effect, which may help you relax and sleep better.

Vegetarianism

For a number of reasons, more and more people are choosing to eat less and less meat. Although some people may eat less because meat is expensive, the majority of decisions are based on current research that indicates that most meat products are just not the healthiest sources of protein.* It is

*See *Eating for the Eighties: a Complete Guide to Vegetarian Nutrition*, and *Jane Brody's Nutrition Book*, listed in the Bibliography.

also a fact that the average American diet is much higher in protein than it needs to be. Meat, high in phosphorus, causes extra calcium to be drawn from the bones to balance the acid level in the blood. This reduced calcium balance contributes to brittle bones later in life. Meat takes longer to digest and can decompose before it's eliminated. When they are cooked, various fats and amino acids in meat produce mutagens and carcinogens. Finally, meat always contains many added growth hormones and antibiotics that are liberally and routinely mixed in with animals' feed (unless the animals are organically raised). Repeated exposure to these substances has already made us more and more resistant to the beneficial effects of the antibiotics that have been created to protect us!

Most people who have decided to change their meat-eating habits are choosing a kind of semivegetarian diet. Although they have not completely cut out meat, they have drastically reduced or eliminated their intake of red meat and have increased their consumption of nonmeat protein sources.

The case for eating less—or no—meat can be made on many grounds other than that of health. However, as in any aspect of yoga practice, the decision to become a partial or total vegetarian should not be forced. To a yogi, health reasons are secondary to the idea of nonviolence. Nonviolence is the first of the *yamas* and *niyamas* (see Chapter 11), ethical guidelines for a life-style that complements the yogi's goals for health and self-awareness. The concept of nonviolence includes not only refraining from harming living creatures but also from harming oneself. It is important to keep this in mind if you begin to change your diet. To start out being vegetarian by forcing yourself before you truly want the change is self-violence! So if you choose to reduce or cut out meat from your diet, do it gradually, and with awareness. Educate yourself about other sources of protein and about protein complementarity (see Suggested Reading).

Once you stop eating meat, it would be an excellent idea to keep track of your meal composition for several days and count the grams of protein you are getting to be sure you are getting enough. Almost every food contains some protein. But only animal sources and a very few vegetable sources are "complete" proteins, meaning that they have some of each of the essential amino acids that comprise proteins. However, a *varied* and *balanced* diet will provide adequate protein over the course of a day from many sources, both singly and in combination.

There are several types of vegetarian diets: the lacto-ovo-vegetarian, which means that one eats dairy products and eggs; the lacto-vegetarian, which means that one eats dairy products but not eggs; the vegan, with no dairy products at all; and the fruitarian, composed only of "fallen fruits," so that no plant has to be killed in the harvesting process. The macrobiotic diet is similar to the vegan, but foods are eliminated in a strictly prescribed progression until, in the ultimate aim of the diet, every category of food except rice is eliminated.

Obviously, the latter three types of vegetarian diets will be much more difficult to maintain and are not recommended. These types of diet can be dangerous because they do not provide several essential nutrients, which must then be supplemented carefully. Besides, unless your major priority in life is monitoring this type of diet, you will have to spend too much of your precious time just finding and preparing the right food to eat. After all, one of the advantages of being a human is that we have learned to anticipate and store our food supplies so that we can spend most of our time on other activities! The stresses, desires and obligations of complex social worlds and abundance of opportunities of the typical American life-style cry out for a balanced approach to all aspects of day-to-day life that will keep you from becoming distracted from your most important goals.

But only you can decide how many of your decisions about what to do and what to eat and how to live should be absolute, firm and unshakable, and how much should be open to occasional variations. It's the position of your mind that is important. How much of your precious energy do you wish to spend on the various aspects of your diet? Many people, trying to be *too* strict with themselves at first, tend to "binge" on the forbidden foods more often because the pressure for perfection is too high. Be careful not to use your diet as an asceticism that punishes more than it supports.

It is important, in the beginning, to allow yourself some outlet for emotional release. Yoga gradually orders the body and the mind into a greater awareness of what causes our different physical, emotional and mental reactions, and then shows us how we can choose to change those reactions so that they conform to our vision of who and what we want to be. (That is *real* freedom, in the yogi's opinion—to be able to choose how we will react to our world!) There is often an unconscious resistance to that change, because change always involves an element of risk, of the unknown.

So, as you begin to build your self-control by doing regular exercise, breathing and meditation; and learn to eat foods that reinforce that growth rather than hinder it, don't ignore that unconscious resistance—it won't go away by itself! You must learn to keep your sense of humor and playfulness intact and allow occasional deviations from your ideal in some areas. Whether you decide to become vegetarian or simply develop the particular healthier eating habits that work for you, monitor your deviations, if you can, and you may learn some valuable lessons about how your mind and emotions work.

Choosing Healthy Alternatives to Processed and Refined Foods

It is interesting and alarming that the Industrial Revolution has run away with us to the extent that we are now processing and refining so many of our good whole foods. The blessing of food preservation has turned into a curse, because so many preservatives and other additives have been found to be harmful. Unfortunately, children who grow up watching enticing commercials and giving in to clever store packaging for sugary foods, artificial treats and other nonfoods develop such a taste for them that they realize only too late—when faced with diabetes, high blood pressure, high cholesterol, heart disease and other illnesses late in life—that they should have changed their eating habits long ago. School lunches offer fried and fatty foods; limp, unappetizing vegetables; soggy white bread and sick-sweet desserts.

If you are concerned about your own and your family's health and wish to start offering healthier alternatives, you will need patience, tact and a certain quality of sneakiness. If your family is used to refined white bread, first switch to a white bread with a couple of extras such as oatmeal or wheat germ. Then try a variety that is mostly white but partly whole wheat. Over time, as tastes change along with the new products, you will be able to move in the direction of 100 percent whole wheat. Experiment with several different brands. Combine white pasta with whole wheat, spinach, tomato,

carrot and other new varieties of pasta. Combine white rice with brown, and be creative with herbs and spices so that the flavors are enhanced. Try new grains such as barley, bulgur, millet and so on, mixed with pasta or rice.

For protein alternatives, try the many different ways of cooking with tofu (soybean curd). Once a fad food, tofu is now found in most supermarkets and is low-cost, low-fat and very versatile. Tofu has no taste of its own and so can be made into an international assortment of flavors and textures. Tofu is also a good egg substitute, since it has very little fat. Other excellent sources of protein are dried beans and peas. Not restricted to dull rice and

beans, legume dishes can be attractive and delicious without being time-consuming to prepare. (See Bibliography for cookbooks that are full of great ideas.)

Fresh fruits and vegetables are better than frozen or canned if you eat them right away. Canned foods always come out lowest in nutrient value, but frozen foods sometimes are higher than fresh, because modern processing is done faster. Fresh foods that sit on the shelf or in your refrigerator for days have lost their chief advantage of being fresh. Nevertheless, even frozen foods can't always compare to the texture and taste of fresh. If you shop once a week, it might be a good idea to use your fresh produce the first

FOOD CRAVINGS

What sounds good to you right at this moment? An apple? A dish of ice cream? A plate of spaghetti? Sometimes your body can tell you what it needs to eat, but sometimes we mistake needs for cravings. For example, when you think you are craving sweets, your body is really saying that it needs energy. The best way to supply that energy is not with sweets, which cause high and low swings in blood sugar, but with foods containing protein and B vitamins (more on that later). As you become more proficient in your yoga practice and more observant of yourself, you'll soon be able to use your "body talk" exercise to make sure you are eating the right things. Can you imagine being able to stand in front of the refrigerator and asking your body to tell you what it needs—and having it say *broccoli!* with glee, instead of *chocolate ice cream*? It does hap-

pen! Rather than having to give up certain foods, you will find that those foods will give *you* up, almost automatically, as your body becomes healthier. They will simply lose their attractiveness to you, and you will happily go on to foods that taste better and make you feel better. You will have successfully translated an emotional or physical need into the right fuel requirement.

Some cravings are so strong they are like true addictions: Caffeine, for example, is a substance on which your body can become dependent—so much so that you will experience withdrawal symptoms of headaches, fatigue and irritability if you try to stop "cold turkey." Caffeine is a stimulant that revs up your body just like regular doses of a commanding stressor. Some people even become addicted to sugar, because of their body's lack of proper en-

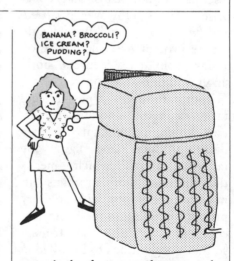

ergy. And, of course, there are alcohol, and drugs, and smoking, all of which rob the body of necessary nutrients. Whatever the addiction, many of our students have found that a balanced diet, with above-average supplies of all nutrients, especially the B and C vitamins, can bring the body up to a healthy state and provide buffers to help with the difficult process of withdrawal.

part of the week and the frozen for the latter part. Experiment with the many varieties of fruits and vegetables. A widely varied diet will give you more essential nutrients than a narrow and limited one. Besides, there are so many new varieties of produce, and the availability of seasonal produce is increasing so fast, it is a shame not to take advantage of the abundance.

If you are trying to cut down on caffeine, try the many available alternatives. Both tea and coffee come in decaffeinated form, although there is controversy over whether the chemicals used in the decaffeination process leave a harmful residue. If you are concerned, brands processed with water only are available from specialty stores. There are also a number of interesting herbal teas available, and herbal "coffee substitutes" that contain no coffee at all. Offer children fruit juice concentrate diluted with plain club soda for a fizzy alternative to carbonated soft drinks.

Sugar substitutes are a problem. All the chemical substitutes now used in commercial products have some health drawbacks. The best solution is simply to cut down on sugar, period. Use less in baked goods, substitute fruit juices or dried fruits, and if you buy canned fruit, use the brands packed in water rather than syrup. Buy cereals with little or no added sweeteners. After a short while your sweet tooth really will become less demanding.

FOOD SUPPLEMENTS

Always a controversial issue, food supplements should be studied carefully by each individual. There are advantages and disad- vantages to supplementing your diet. If you have doubts or questions, read extensively and consult with a qualified physician or nutritionist. In the American Yoga Association classes, we briefly discuss nutrition as part of the regular curriculum, with an emphasis on commonsense information about eating more healthfully as part of a yogic life-style. These recommendations should not be construed as professional medical or dietary advice.

While it may be true that a person can get all of his or her neces- sary vitamins and minerals from food, it is hardly likely that most people eat so carefully or so much. In this country we place such a high value on thinness that many of us are constantly "watching our weight" and for that reason eat erratically and poorly. Furthermore, the prevalence of highly refined and processed foods makes it even less likely that our daily diet contains adequate amounts of necessary nutrients. Some nutritionists believe that many people live on the edge of malnutrition, exhibiting

FOOD AND ILLNESS

When you are under stress, or when you are depressed or anxious, your immune system does not function as well as when you are feeling better. Researchers have noted that people who feel loved and cared for get sick less often than people who feel lonely or abandoned much of the time. Perhaps it is because yoga helps improve your self-image, your management of stress and your feelings of well-being that people who practice yoga generally seem to become more resistant to infection and seem to recover from illness faster.

A proper diet can also help you resist letting illness into your body. A diet fortified in the infection-fighting nutrients—vitamins C and A—and consisting of a variety of whole foods can build strong resistance to infection.

If you do get sick, use your common sense and follow your doctor's advice. Drink plenty of fluids, and follow your body's direction about how much to eat. Don't practice your yoga asans, because you might spread the infection, especially with upside-down poses. Do give yourself some extra rest time. Illness is a powerful stressor. Don't push yourself to work when your body is saying that it needs rest. Perhaps you could catch up on some books you've been wanting to read, or spend some extra time with meditation.

If you have head or chest congestion, you may find it helpful to cut way down on dairy products. Drink lots of sweet and salty liquids, such as fruit juice, herb tea and soup. Don't force your body to eat more than it wants to eat; sometimes, such as when you have a fever, your body will naturally want to reduce its food intake in order to "starve out" the infecting viruses. Many of our students have found it helpful to increase their vitamin C intake for short periods of time when they feel an infection coming on; powdered ascorbic acid melted and mixed with juice is more quickly absorbed than tablets. Extra calcium and B vitamins, together with adequate protein and vitamin A, may also help your body get back to health more easily.

enough symptoms of various kinds to feel less than 100 percent fit and healthy but not sick enough to see a doctor. Food supplements cannot and should not be used to replace food, but a daily multivitamin and mineral supplement most likely will not harm you and may provide that extra "edge" that ensures against deficiency and illness. Some vitamins (particularly A and D) and minerals can be toxic in large doses, so be sure to find a brand that does not offer therapeutic amounts, unless that amount has been recommended by your doctor or nutritionist.*

If you are on special medications, you will have to be extra careful. Some medications make nutrient deficiencies worse; however, some nutrient supplements may also counteract the effects of the medication. For example, large amounts of aspirin can interfere with iron absorption. Diuretics deplete calcium, potassium and magnesium. Antibiotics reduce many nutrients because they kill all bacteria, not just the harmful ones, and many nutrients are produced by beneficial bacteria in the body. However, acidic foods such as fruit juices can interfere with the effectiveness of the antibiotic. If you are in doubt, check with your doctor.

Some foods such as nutritional yeast are used successfully by many students to provide an extra

*The Vitamin Bible, by Earl Mindell, listed in the Bibliography, is a good source for recommended amounts of nutrients.

"energy boost" during the day without a lot of extra calories. Nutritional yeast is a powdered or flaked food grown especially for nutritional purposes (it is not baking yeast) and is similar to brewer's yeast but less strong-tasting. Nutritional yeast provides balanced B-complex vitamins, some protein and a little fat, making it an ideal snack. It has the added advantage of being filling, so that you are less likely to overeat on less nutritious snacks. Start small if you are adding nutritional yeast to your diet—take one teaspoon in juice or water twice daily. Some people notice gas or bloating the first week, which is natural if the body is not used to it. Gradually work up to one or two tablespoons at a time. Taking yeast tablets is not recommended. Not only are many people allergic to the fillers used in the tablets, but also, because of the extra fillers and binders, you would have to take a great many tablets to equal a tablespoon of powder. If you are taking two or more tablespoons of yeast daily, and/or you are not a vegetarian, make sure that you are getting enough calcium, as the phosphorus in the yeast (as in all protein) must be balanced with calcium.

Calcium is a mineral that is receiving much more attention, as authorities continue to study the correlations between low calcium intake and the development of osteoporosis in later years. Most current authorities agree that the old standard of 800 milligrams is not enough and that daily intake should be more like 1000 milli-

grams and perhaps higher for some women.* Consider a calcium supplement if your intake from food is low. Foods high in calcium: dairy products, tofu, dark green leafy vegetables, oysters.

If you choose not to take a daily multivitamin/mineral supplement, you might at least consider the following suggested "stress formula" of a few separate vitamins, to take once or twice daily with a meal. This combination replaces the nutrients lost most readily in our many daily stress reactions:

- B complex, timed-release form —at least 10 mg of B_1, B_2, B_6
- C, timed-release form—100-500 mg, plus bioflavanoids (aids absorption)
- Calcium—about 500 mg, or according to your dietary intake. It is important to have adequate vitamin D for absorption of calcium, and many nutritionists believe that magnesium is also important in this role. Many calcium supplements include these two nutrients. Do not use bone meal or dolomite for calcium supplementation because of their possible high lead content
- Nutritional yeast (not baking yeast!)—which also includes protein and B vitamins. Start with 1 teaspoon twice daily with meals; work up to 2 tablespoons

*Dawson-Hughes, Bess, "How Diet Can Help Prevent Brittle Bones," in Tufts University Diet and Nutrition Letter, Vol. I, No. 3, May 1983.

CHAPTER 8
YOGA DURING PREGNANCY

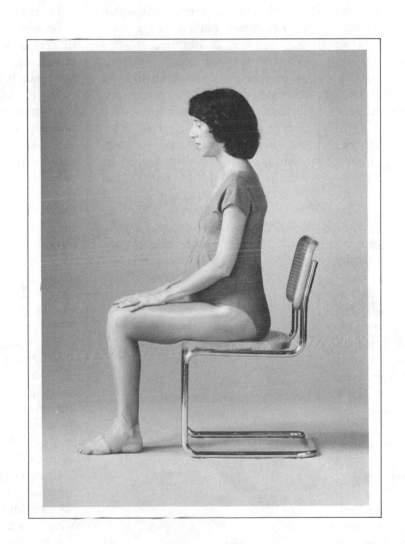

During pregnancy, you and your body have a very special relationship. You are both working together for one purpose, which overrides all others: producing a healthy baby. Instinctively your body knows what to do; and yoga can help you support this special work.

The objectives for maintaining a yoga routine during the last six months of pregnancy are primarily to improve relaxation skills. This training will help you relieve lower back pain and postural tension as your carriage changes with weight gain, and will improve your concentration and relaxation for labor and delivery. The simple routines also help strengthen your nervous system and increase joint limberness and strength. Naturally, if you have started a yoga routine before your pregnancy, you will have an easier time maintaining it throughout your term, and the benefits will increase.

If you are planning to become pregnant, you can give yourself and your baby a head start by working on improving your health. Begin right away to improve your diet, get enough rest, learn techniques to help manage your stress and practice yoga exercises to build stability in your nervous system, strength in your lower back and abdomen, improved circulation in your legs and increased joint limberness. Practice all these suggestions regularly, and by the time you get pregnant, they will have become second nature, and it will be that much easier to motivate yourself to continue.

As soon as you suspect that you are pregnant, stop doing any yoga exercises at all, and don't resume until the first trimester (first three months) has passed, assuming there have been no complications

and your doctor approves. The reasons for this caution are, first of all, that in the first few months of pregnancy your body is working hard to establish a new hormone balance, and the strong effects that yoga exercises have on the hormonal system might obstruct or counteract this natural change. Second, the compression involved in many yoga exercises might exacerbate any existing problems of which you may or may not be aware.

After the first three months you may resume a modified yoga exercise routine as outlined in this chapter. If your doctor suggests maintaining an alternate form of exercise during your pregnancy, discuss the best possibilities with him or her; perhaps a mildly aerobic workout such as walking, swimming or bicycling would be best. Most women are encouraged to keep up their regular levels of daily activity. However, keep in mind that starting a new exercise activity that is foreign to your body is not usually recommended in the middle of pregnancy.

HELPFUL HINTS

As you practice your medically approved routine during the second and third trimester, do only what is comfortable. You may find it increasingly difficult toward the end of your term to motivate yourself to exercise. Don't force it, but do try to incorporate some of the techniques into other activities, such as supported leg lifts while working in the kitchen, or shoulder and neck rotations while reading.

Because of the increased levels of certain hormones during pregnancy, your joints will naturally become a bit looser. Be careful not to injure yourself: Pay attention to your kinesthetic sense (the awareness of where your body is in space) and move deliberately and slowly. If you normally run or participate in other vigorous exercise (and your doctor approves of continuing), be even more careful than usual so that your increased looseness does not result in a fall. Be aware that your center of gravity is changing also, and guard against the falls that can be caused by this physical change. Hold on to a sturdy chair or counter when doing standing exercises.

Breathing techniques can be done in any comfortable seated position. Use one or more pillows for extra height if you sit on the floor, in order to reduce strain on the lower back. You may also sit on the edge of a chair for breathing (see page 165 and Chapter 5 for more suggestions on proper posture and seat for breathing.) Many women find that yoga practice complements Lamaze training because of the emphasis on paced, focused breathing.

Many women report that meditation during pregnancy becomes more difficult as their mental strength is drawn even further inward to fuel the unconscious bodily functions necessary for the development of the baby. Some women describe the feeling as a warm woolen cap fitted over their brain! It becomes much more difficult to disengage your conscious mind from this unconscious process as the pregnancy develops. If this happens to you, shift your attention from achieving a quietness or detachment in meditational experience to more work on the experience of complete physical and mental relaxation. Use the relaxation procedure as taught, but make it a process that you employ for the whole session. Concentrate on problem areas such as the face, the stomach and the shoulders, and focus on increasing your ability to spot tension and relax it at will. This training will help your concentration and ability to relax as you go into labor. A welcome plus is that the more happy, calm and relaxed you are, the more happy and relaxed your baby will be.

Practice your relaxation/meditation lying down, or sitting with your back leaning against a straight chair or the wall, or seated with crossed legs. Experiment with one or more pillows under or between your knees, under your lower back or under your head for additional comfort. You can lie on your side with a pillow under your head, one between your knees, and perhaps even another under the side of your stomach. Any position that is comfortable for you is the position you should use.

YOGA ROUTINE FOR PREGNANCY

Many of the exercises you may do have already been illustrated elsewhere in this book. *Never* do any inverted (upside-down) positions when you are pregnant because of the danger of air embolism. Compression poses are also not recommended, except for the Baby Pose and the Diamond Pose. Exercises described previously are listed along with their page numbers; new exercises* are illustrated on the following pages:

Arm Rolls, p. 23
Neck Stretch, p. 24
Shoulder Shrug, p. 21
Elbow Touch, p. 22
Easy Bend, p. 27
Full Bend, p. 28 (Hold on to chair with one hand, letting the other arm relax. Do not stretch too far down in this exercise, to guard against hyperextending the spine.)
*Supported Leg Lifts, p. 164
*Baby Pose, p. 164
Cat Breath, p. 74
*Pelvic Rock, p. 165
Foot Flaps, p. 86
Diamond Pose, p. 95
Easy Twist (cross-legged), p. 91
Easy Bridge, p. 52
Alternate Toe Touch, p. 101 (through the 7th month only.)

Following is a suggested six-week course progression:

WEEK ONE:
Complete Breath, standing
Arm Rolls
Neck Stretch
Easy Bend
Baby Pose
Relaxation and Meditation

WEEK TWO, ADD:
Full Bend (if allowed)
Foot Flap
Diamond Pose and Warm-up
Humming Breath

WEEK THREE, ADD:
Standing Reach without arm stretch (hold on to chair with both hands instead)
Sit-Between-Feet (see following)
Pelvic Rock
Standing Leg Lifts

WEEK FOUR, ADD:
Easy Spine Twist
Easy Bridge

WEEKS FIVE AND SIX:
Continue same routine

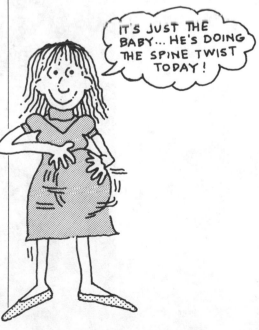

IT'S JUST THE BABY... HE'S DOING THE SPINE TWIST TODAY!

SUPPORTED LEG LIFTS

Stand beside a chair, holding on to the back for support. Stare at one spot on the wall in front of you for additional help with balance. Keep breath relaxed. Lift the leg about three times forward (A), then to the side (B), then back (C). Keep foot flexed at all times to strengthen legs and increase circulation.

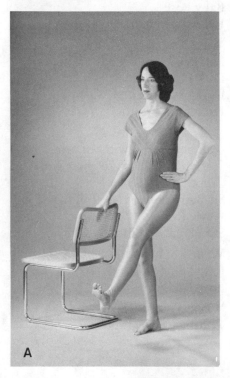

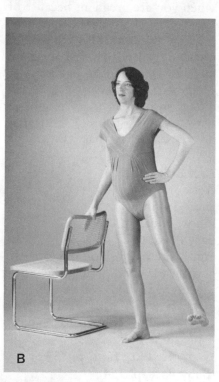

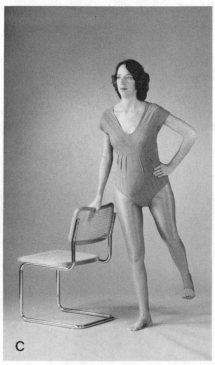

BABY POSE

(A) Separate knees a foot or more —as far as is necessary as your abdomen increases in size. If discomfort results from your head being below your heart, rest your head on your arms as shown instead of bending your arms back toward the feet as shown earlier in this book. If this pose becomes too uncomfortable (this is a normal occurrence), just relax for a few minutes in your favorite rest position.

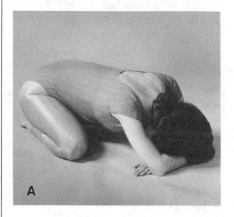

PELVIC ROCK

(A–B) This exercise, shown kneeling, can also be done standing or seated on feet. Its purpose is to strengthen and relieve tension in the lower back. Kneel with back straight. Exhale, pulling your lower back and stomach in, making a straighter back, without slouching. Then breathe in, letting stomach relax, and arch the lower back forward (this movement is similar to the Cat Breath). Repetitions: 3.

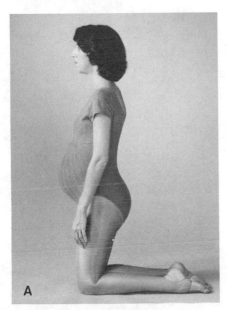

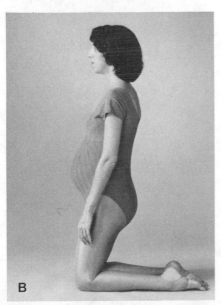

BREATHING

For your breathing routine, practice sitting between your feet (A) on one or more pillows to limber hips and knees. Any seated poses on the floor are recommended for promoting flexibility and joint strength. Sit on the floor while watching television, reading or playing with other children in the family. The Complete Breath is your best technique for stress reduction and breath control at any time of day. It can be done standing, sitting, kneeling or lying down. The Complete Breath can also be an effective sleep aid. The Humming Breath is a good focusing exercise to change mood or relax jittery emotions. Use the Laughasan to relax facial muscles and change mood.

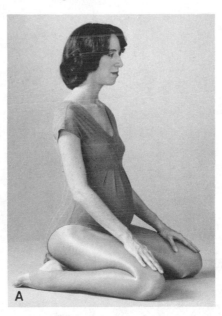

DIET AND NUTRITION

Before you get pregnant, give your baby a healthy start by developing new, healthier eating habits yourself. Stop smoking. Reduce or eliminate caffeine, sugar, food additives and excess fat. Eliminate alcohol. The following are a few suggestions, but if you are unsure about how to plan an adequate diet, consult your doctor or a registered dietician for advice.

Make sure you are eating a balanced and varied diet, especially adequate in the B vitamins. (See Chapter 7 for the suggestions on good Nutrition, and Suggested Reading section to find out where to go for more information on nutrition during pregnancy.) An adequate supply of balanced B vitamins in your diet may help reduce the incidence of morning sickness.

As your baby grows, many of your organs, including the stomach, are subjected to extra pressure. If it is uncomfortable for you to eat large meals, start eating several smaller meals instead. This has advantages and disadvantages. The advantage is that it helps your body fight stress, because you are frequently replenishing the nutrients used in the stress reactions. A disadvantage is that you have to be very careful to plan all your meals so that you don't end up eating several convenient but nonnutritive snacks that just add empty calories. Six small high-protein meals are recommended.

After the baby is born, if you decide to nurse you should again reduce the amount of exercise you do. Because of their effects on the glandular system, which dictates the composition of the milk, only the following yoga techniques should be done while nursing:

Arm Rolls
Neck Stretch
Tree Pose
Sit-Between-Feet
Complete Breath
Relaxation and Meditation

CHAPTER 9
YOGA AND SPORTS

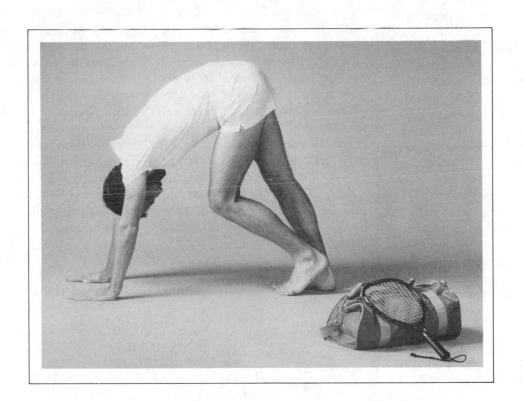

Contrary to what you might expect, the slow, controlled, relaxed movements of yoga asans can be complementary to active sports. In fact, they may even help improve your performance!

HOW ASANS HELP

By doing a yoga asan routine every day, you will build a reserve of flexibility and strength that keeps you in shape, allowing you to exercise more often, stay fresher and recover faster. Yoga can also help by balancing the muscle groups that are being overlooked in your favorite sport. Strength/flexibility imbalances are the greatest cause of injury. In running, for example, you will strengthen the muscles in the back of your legs, but without stretching exercises, the muscles will tighten more and more. This chapter will give you a general routine to keep you in shape every day, plus suggestions for different types of stretches that work best for different sports.

HOW BREATHING HELPS

Don't forget to practice breathing exercises to enhance your sports activities. Practice in breathing can increase your stamina. The Belly Breath is especially helpful because it teaches you how to keep your stomach muscles relaxed *while you are exercising*, which can help prevent side stitch. Using breath before competition can focus your mind and increase your concentration.

HOW RELAXATION AND MEDITATION HELP

A daily practice of yoga relaxation and meditation can train you to be more aware of your body so that you can relax the muscles you don't need to use. If you are competitive, relaxation training can help you cope with precompeti-tion anxiety so that your performance is not hampered.

USING YOGA FOR WARMING UP AND COOLING DOWN

Whether you are a competitive athlete or just follow an every-other-day aerobics workout to condition your heart and lungs, you can benefit from using yoga asans to help you warm up and cool down.

Just as in preparation for a yoga routine, warming up is essential. Warming up is a way of telling your body that you are about to demand more work from it. If you and your body work as a team rather than at odds, you will both enjoy your activities a lot more. Learn your body's weak points, its likes and dislikes, its fears and comfort levels, and you can gently coax it along to achieve your athletic goals. You can get more out of your body, with fewer complaints, if you take the time to understand and work with its characteristics rather than forcing it with the idea of "whipping into shape." Make friends with your body—don't become its slave driver.

Many experts agree that the "static" or relaxed holding stretches of yoga are ideal for warming up before and cooling down after a strenuous workout and actually work better than the bouncy, "ballistic" stretches that many inexperienced athletes use. This is because muscles automatically contract when they are stretched near their limit, in an instinctive reaction to avoid being torn. If the stretch is held, the muscle gradually relaxes and is able to stretch even farther without injury. However, if the muscle is pushed to its limit by quick bounces, it retains the contraction and is much more vulnerable to tearing, both in the stretch routine and in the workout.

Cooling down after your workout is just as important as warming up beforehand. Many people who allocate adequate warm-up time tend to leave out or skimp on cooling-down time. While it is true that your body can eventually recover by itself, it will take much longer and be harder on your system than it would be if you spent a few minutes helping the process along.

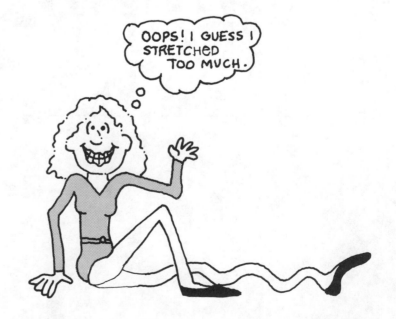

During a workout your muscles contract and your blood pressure naturally rises as your heart pumps faster in order to supply the muscle cells and tissues with needed oxygen. If you end your workout abruptly, your muscles stop contracting; less blood is pumped through the heart, and your blood pressure falls rapidly. A possible result is the pooling of blood in the extremities, especially the legs, causing still-needed oxygen to be less available to the muscles. In addition, you may experience dizziness, nausea or lightheadedness.

To avoid these symptoms, keep moving for a few minutes after a workout—walk around awhile, and then start some stretches to keep the blood delivering oxygen to cells and tissues, flush out metabolic wastes and start any cell repair work. First stretch the muscles that were used the hardest during your workout, and then end with generalized stretches.

Following are a few suggestions for using the exercises described earlier in this book—along with some new ones—to help you get the most from your sports activities. If you like, add one of the specialized routines for individual sports to the general, daily sports routine.

DAILY YOGA ROUTINE FOR IMPROVED SPORTS PERFORMANCE

V-RAISE WITH BENT LEG

In the V-Raise position, head tucked and legs straight, bend one leg and put your weight on the straight leg, pressing your heel toward the floor to stretch the back of the leg. Hold for a few seconds, breathing gently, then repeat on opposite side.

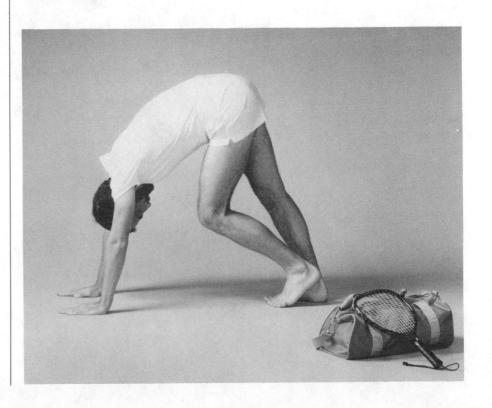

90-DEGREE STRETCH

In a seated position with legs out-stretched, bend left leg back to the left with your toes curled around your hip. Stretch your thigh as far as possible—eventually you want your left thigh to be perpendicular to your outstretched right leg. Now lean back on your elbows (A), or as far as possible, and hold, breathing gently, for several seconds. If you are very limber, you may be able to lie completely back (B). Repeat on opposite side.

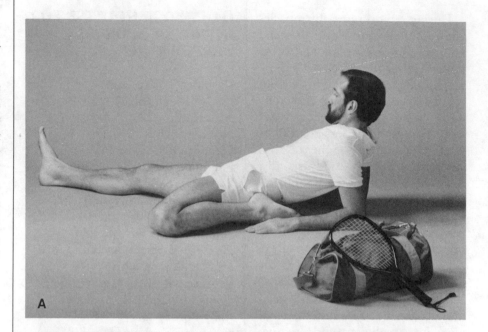

A

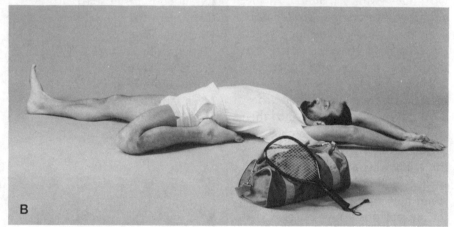

B

LUNGE

With feet apart a comfortable distance, toes pointed inward, bend gently toward the right, placing your fists on either side of your right foot; your right fist will actually be in *back* of the right foot with your lifted elbow tucked under your bent knee (A). Hold the position for a few seconds, breathing gently. Repeat on left side. After you can do this without strain, try lifting your back knee off the floor (B). To intensify the stretch even more, and to extend the stretch to the groin muscles, bend farther toward the floor so that you are resting on your elbows (C) instead of your fists.

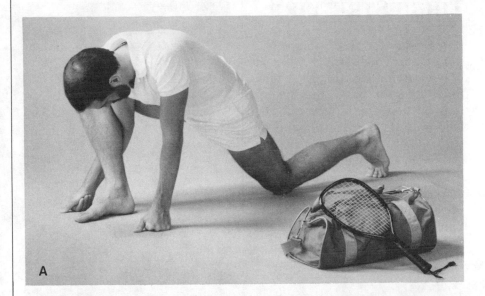

A

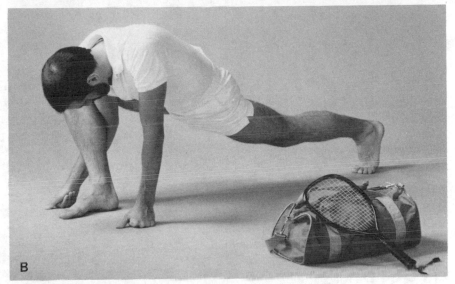

B

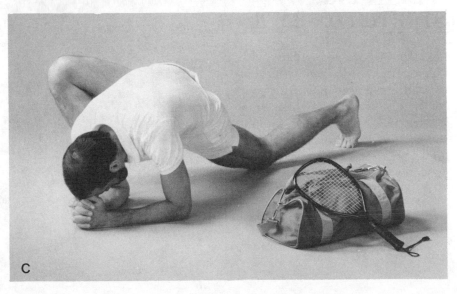

C

THIGH STRETCH II

Instructions for II: In this variation to the Thigh Stretch, start in Thigh Stretch position but tuck toes under in back. Breathe in, look up and stretch forward, lifting the back knee off the floor (A); then breathe out and straighten *both* legs, tucking your head toward your front leg as far as possible, and pushing the heel of your back leg down toward the floor (B). Repetitions: 3 on each side.

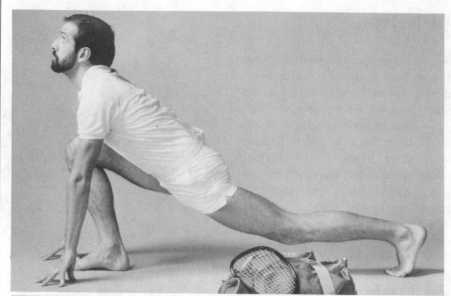

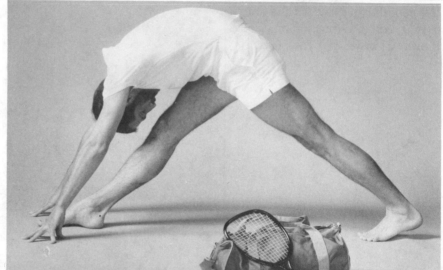

HAMSTRING STRETCH ON BACK

Leaning on your right elbow with legs outstretched, bend your left leg and grasp your toes with your left hand. Slowly straighten your left leg as far as possible without strain, and hold for several seconds, breathing normally. Repeat on opposite side.

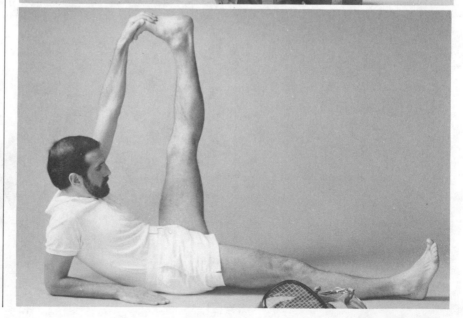

Special Help from Yoga for Your Favorite Sport

FOR BICYCLING

(to stretch the chest and stomach backward, and to strengthen lower back)

Add
Side Triangle (p. 60)
T-Pose with Knee Bends (p. 69)
Camel Pose (p. 82)
Cobra Pose (p. 121)
Alternate Arm and Leg Balance (p. 73)
Pigeon Pose (p. 84)

FOR RACQUETBALL, TENNIS, ETC.

(to strengthen knees and lower back, stretch inner thigh, improve respiration and improve range of motion of the shoulder)

Add
T-Pose with Knee Bends (p. 69)
Side Triangle (p. 60)
Twisting Triangle (p. 61)
Full Triangle (p. 58)
Hero Pose Variation (p. 79)
Sun Pose Variation (p. 72)
Easy Balance Twist (p. 55)
Bow Variation (p. 76)
Airplane Series (p. 118)

FOR WEIGHT LIFTING

(to stretch all muscle groups, especially the back of the legs, chest and stomach, and upper and lower back)

Add
Full Triangle (p. 58)
Side Triangle (p. 60)
Twisting Triangle (p. 61)
Lunge (p. 171)
Pigeon Pose (p. 84)
Seated Sun Pose (p. 86)
Alternate Seated Sun Pose (p. 89)
Cobra Pose (p. 121)
Spine Twist (p. 179)
Pelvic Twist (p. 103)

Bow Pose (p. 122)
Plow Pose Variations (p. 113)
Hamstring Stretch on Back (p. 172)

FOR SWIMMING

(to improve range of motion of the shoulder joint, strengthen lower back and stretch upper back and ribs, and improve respiration)

Add
Dancer Pose (p. 66)
Alternate Triangle (p. 59)
Easy Balance Twist (p. 55)
Sun Pose Variation (p. 72)
Side Triangle (p. 60)
Bow Variation (p. 76)
Pigeon Pose (p. 84)
Cobra Pose (p. 121)

FOR GOLF

(to strengthen lower back and improve flexibility of the spine, especially laterally)

Add
Spine Twist (p. 92)
Alternate Triangle (p. 59)
Twisting Triangle (p. 61)
Dancer Pose (p. 66)
Knee Squeeze (p. 179)
Cobra Pose (p. 121)

FOR SKIING

(to strengthen knee joints and lower back, and stretch ankles, thighs and back of calves)

Add
Side Triangle (p. 60)
Cobra V-Raise (p. 77)
Seated Sun Pose (p. 86)
T Pose with Knee Bends (p. 69)
Ankle Stretch (p. 81)
Thigh Stretch II (p. 172)
Pigeon Pose (p. 84)

FOR WALKING AND RUNNING

(to stretch the back of the thigh and calf, top of ankle and front of thigh)

Add
Dancer Pose (p. 66)
Lunge (p. 171)
Thigh Stretch II (p. 172)
Ankle Stretch (p. 81)
Camel Pose (p. 82)
Seated Sun Pose (p. 86)
Alternate Seated Sun Pose (p. 89)
Hamstring Stretch on Back (p. 172)

CHAPTER 10

YOGA FOR STRESS MANAGEMENT

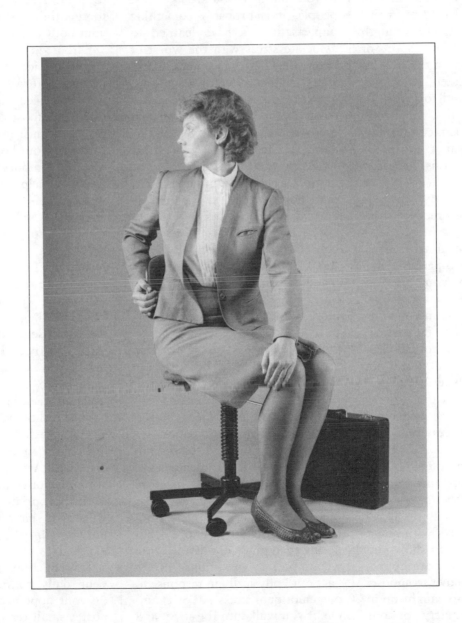

Life is never free from stress, but often it seems that everyone else has less of it than we do. In actual fact, our neighbors may just get stressed by different things then we do or have differing reactions to their stress. Or just maybe, they've learned some techniques to help cope.

It *is* a fact that many people are less negatively affected by stress because of their outlook on life: They have learned that by maintaining their health and strength and by adjusting their point of view, they can look on the stresses of life as challenges and as opportunities to learn and to grow. To such people, no new or unexpected experience is met automatically with despair, anger or dread. Because of this balanced outlook, they are able to reduce the amount of time and effort it takes their bodies to recover from a stress reaction.

If you do not recognize yourself in that description, perhaps this chapter can help you discover ways of changing your personal reactions to the stress in your life. Each person's life has its particular tensions. Some are manageable; some are not. Our aim is not to eliminate the experiences that cause you stress (we can't do very much about that; see Suggested Reading for resources that may help you learn how to reduce the amount of stress in your life), but we *can* do something about changing your *reactions* to stress. For example, if you habitually respond to traffic delays with anger and frustration, we can show you how to substitute a more appropriate and productive response. Sometimes we get so caught up in the what-next? anxiety of our busy lives that it starts to resemble a broken record that buries us ever deeper in hopeless and help-less feelings. Simple yoga techniques applied during the course of a day can put an end to the "broken record" of repeated anxieties, so we end up with more choices and more control in life; so *we* run the show instead of the show running us—into the ground.

When someone mentions *stress*, what is the first thing that comes to your mind? If you are like most people, it is probably something unpleasant. We have learned to associate stress with the worst of everything—pressure at work, short tempers, furrowed brows, antacids, illness and so on. What most people overlook is the fact that stress can be positive, too. Indeed, a life without *any* stress would be dull and boring! A promotion, a wedding, moving into a new home—these happy events are also sources of stress.

The body does not distinguish between "good" stress or "bad" stress. It views all stressors as demands—usually only temporary but sometimes extended—for more work and more energy output.

Recalling a past stress can also create a demand, because the mind signals its original physical reaction as it relives previous feelings of fear, excitement, anger, pain, anxiety and anticipation. It's almost as if we carry a cassette library of events in our memories to replay at will! Even an imagined or anticipated stressor can cause physical reactions. In fact, emotional stressors can be more debilitating than physical ones, because we are socially conditioned not to "act out" physically in response to our emotional stresses. For example, if you walk into the street and see a truck approaching at high speed, your body immediately and automatically responds by quickly getting itself out of the way. Once you are safe, your body's systems soon return to normal. But if you are being yelled at by your boss at work, you may have an intense emotional reaction that you are unable to express and that builds up a great deal of residual internal tension. You may not have the opportunity to express your feelings or to work out the tension physically until much later (if at all), forcing the stress to accumulate in your body and mind.

Earlier in this book we discussed the idea that the body has its own point of view, its own desires and needs, and that in order to get the most out of yoga practice, you must learn to communicate with your body. This becomes especially important when you are trying to help your body become more stress resistant. In this chapter we will show you how to recognize your body's reactions to stress and specific constructive techniques for "working out" and eliminating the debilitating and exhausting physical syndrome. Yoga can help you *recover* from the extra demands of life stresses more quickly and at the same time teach you to *change* your responses to more positive ones. Yoga also can be viewed as a *preventive* technique, enabling you to start out each day with more resistance and more energy at your disposal. After all, why waste your precious energy on negative or inappropriate stress responses when you have better things to do!

Schedule some of the following stress-reduction techniques into your daily routine—mark them on your appointment calendar or post a small reminder above your work station if you think you'll forget. Remember that the effects of yoga are cumulative.

THREE STEPS TO GREATER STRESS RESISTANCE

1. Learn To Recognize Your Body's Particular Signals.

You can help your body cope with the demands of stress by learning to recognize its signals. Here are some examples of various kinds of signals your body may be sending when it is under stress:

a. **physical:** frequent headaches, migraine headaches and symptoms, numbness in extremities, unusual amount of blinking or yawning, rapid heartbeat, rapid breathing, nervous tics, teeth clenching, nausea, insomnia, sighing

b. **perceptual:** losing perspective (making a mountain out of a molehill), repeated forgetfulness, misperceptions (failing to hear or see accurately), inattentiveness or distractibility (daydreaming, poor concentration)

c. **emotional:** blowing up/loss of temper, high or low irritability (either everything or nothing bothers you), unexplained or prolonged depression, crying

d. **behavioral:** nervous habits (tapping, etc.); sudden changes in diet; accident proneness; increased use of alcohol, caffeine, smoking, sugar, etc.

States of mind are often mirrored in the body. Such expressions as Grin and bear it; Keep a stiff upper lip and The strong, silent type are illustrative of the extremely common stress response of tightening facial muscles, especially those of the jaw. Can you see how, in our society, we perpetuate such responses by our attitude toward them? We actually increase these responses by our tacit approval, as revealed in these common expressions. To our great detriment, we have trained ourselves to define self-control as muscle tension and inhibited expression.

Can you think of other expressions that illustrate the way we respond to stress?

He's a pain in the neck. Translation: I tighten my neck and throat muscles to avoid saying how I really feel about him.

I am petrified she's going to get angry with me. Translation: I am so afraid of her response that my brain can't send the right signals to my muscles in order to move correctly, so I feel stiff.

His attitude makes my blood boil. Translation: Since I don't dare tell him what I think of his actions, my emotional reaction to him causes my body to react with increasing blood pressure and pulse rate.

You make me sick! Translation: My interaction with you raises such anxiety that my stomach feels tense and nauseous.

I'm all keyed up about tomorrow's meeting. Translation: My muscles are tight and tense as if to defend me from attack or allow me to run away to safety.

Which parts of *your* body react most quickly to stress? Take a few minutes right now to write down how *your* body reacts to stress.

2. Learn Which Techniques are the Most Effective For Modifying Your Personal Stress Reactions.

Does your body conspire with you in taking your job home at night? All day long you store muscle tension from many sources: staying in one position too long, not being able to express your feelings, sitting with poor posture, being anxious. Your body is not meant to be as inactive as most of ours are. When inactivity is coupled with stored muscle tension, fatigue is compounded. In some ways the increased efficiency of modern office design can perpetuate muscle tension! If you have only to swivel your chair to get from file cabinet to keyboard to telephone to copier to supply shelf to coffee machine, you'll have little cause for movement. And if you combine this essential inactivity with poor air circulation, poorly fitted furniture and consumption of caffeine and sugar, it's no wonder you are tired at the end of the day!

Yoga exercises release stored muscle tension by gently pushing, stretching and compressing muscle tissue, nerves, blood vessels and major organs. By performing a balanced series of movements regularly, you can reduce the amount of tension you take home at the end of the day. Plus, the extra circulation helps get more oxygen and other nutrients to your brain, where they will help wake you up. Sometimes those feelings of sleepiness and lethargy in the late afternoon are simply a result of stiffened neck muscles that reduce circulation to the head.

YOUR BODY'S TARGET ZONES

Following is a list of the major trouble spots for stored tension, and of the yoga techniques that are best for relieving stress in these problem areas, once you have identified your own. (See p. 181 for an all-around routine that combines a little of each of these four sets of techniques.) Most of the exercises indicated here are taught earlier in this book in standing or kneeling positions; however, they can be done just as easily in a straight chair. If your feet can't rest flat on the floor, put a book under them.

Did you know that you can use water to change the way you feel? Before you eat, wash your hands and sprinkle some water on your face, concentrating on "washing away" any anxieties, upsets or issues that may be pressing on you. After work (or at least sometime before bedtime) take a warm shower or bath. The warmth will help relax your muscles, and you can imagine the water also rinsing away the troubles and tensions that cling to you each day.

In mythology, water is often used to symbolize a change in consciousness. Many ancient and modern rituals employ this concept (e.g., Christian baptism, the Jewish mikvah, etc.). On a daily basis we often get so caught up in the petty details and little crises in our lives that we forget the things that are really important to us. Water can be a daily reminder to broaden our outlook so that we don't waste our energies on minor, unnecessarily stressful details that don't really matter in the long run.

1 Neck/Upper Back—Shoulder Rolls (p. 21), Elbow Touch (p. 22), Neck Stretch (p. 24), Arm Rolls (p. 23), Standing Reach (p. 26), Easy Bend (p. 27)

Poor posture, keyboard work, sitting in one position too long—all fatigue the muscles in the upper back and neck, causing them to react by tensing. Often this cuts off circulation to the head, which can result in tension headaches. Poor lighting or eye strain can cause us to hunch forward to try to see better. **If you have frequent or severe pain in your neck or upper back, consult a physician before attempting any of these exercises.**

2 Lower Back—Back Arch (p. 134), Folded Pose (p. 179), Knee Squeeze (pp. 32, 99 or 179), Full Bend (p. 28), Cat Breath (p. 74)

Work that requires a lot of standing or bending, poorly fitted furniture that does not support the lower back, as well as pathological problems—slipped, swollen, herniated or degenerating disks—can cause aches and pains in the lower back. Lower back and hip inactivity can also contribute to lack of circulation and stiffness in the legs. **If you have frequent or severe pain in your back, consult a physician before attempting any of these exercises.**

3 Face/jaw/temple—Lion (p. 139), Meditation (p. 148), Neck Stretch (p. 24), Folded Pose (p. 179)

There are thousands of tiny muscles in our faces, which help us produce so many varieties of facial expressions; yet they also tighten up easily, especially if you are a "teeth clencher"! Sometimes headaches can result from this continual tension, which constricts the blood vessels in your head, thus causing them to "rebound" by dilating, which causes the pain. **Note: If you often get pain in your temples, cheekbones and bridge of nose, you may have a chronic sinus condition. Frequent or severe pain in your temples or on one or both sides of your head—sometimes accompanied by visual or other unusual symptoms—may indicate migraine. Consult a physician for either condition before attempting any exercises.**

4 Stomach/Chest—Belly Breath (p. 136), Back Arch (p. 134), Seated Twist (p. 179), Cat Breath (p. 74), Folded Pose (p. 179)

This area is probably the most important of all. Tensing the muscles of your stomach, abdomen and rib cage prevents you from breathing deeply and completely. As you have probably read already in Chapter 5 on breath, there is a direct connection between the degree of relaxation of your breath and the state of your emotions. **Note: Tightness in your chest or a feeling of pressure is a common stress response but also can be an indicator of heart trouble in some individuals. If you experience this sensation often or severely, consult your physician immediately.**

Most of these exercises are described previously in standing or kneeling positions, and most can be done seated just as they are done standing. A couple of exceptions are:

SEATED SPINE TWIST

Sit forward on the chair, with feet flat on the floor. Place your right hand on your left knee, and your left arm over the back of the chair or just in front of the chair back. Hold on to back, side or seat of chair (experiment to find the best grip for you.) Look forward and breathe in, then slowly breathe out and turn toward your left, pulling with both hands enough to twist your spine as far as possible without strain (A). Hold for a few seconds, breathing easily. Then return to the front and switch sides. Repetitions: 1 to 3 each side.

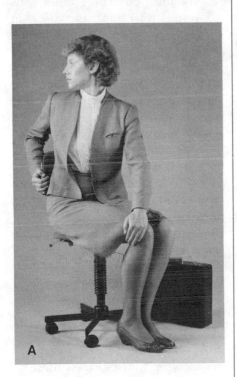

A

SEATED KNEE SQUEEZE

Sit forward on the chair, with feet flat and arms hanging at your sides. Breathe out, then breathe in and lift your right knee up toward your face. Grasp the knee with both hands and hold your breath in while squeezing the knee toward your chest as far as possible (B). Now release and breathe out, and return the leg to the floor. If you have injured or arthritic knees, grasp your thigh just behind the knee instead. Repetitions: 3 on each side.

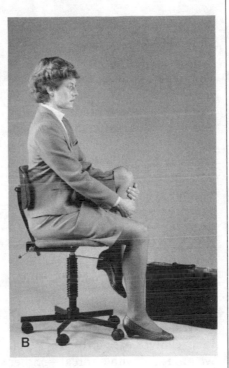

B

FOLDED POSE

Sit with hips touching the back of the chair and feet flat. If your feet don't reach the floor, put a book under them. Separate your knees slightly. Lean forward, using your hands on your knees as a support. If comfortable, rest your chest on your knees, letting your head hang between your knees and your arms hang down at your sides or rest on your feet (C). If this position is not comfortable, cross your arms on your knees and rest your head on your arms. Let your breath relax.

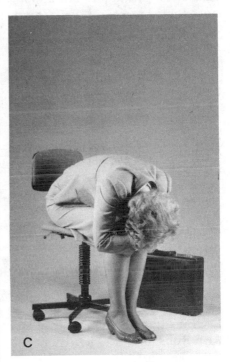

C

3. Make Time Every Day To Put The Techniques Into Practice.

ANYTIME ROUTINES

Doing yoga techniques at any time of day will help reduce the effects of accumulated muscle tension before they turn into unpleasant results such as headache and stomach upset. Nobody has to know that you're doing these exercises! Make it a challenge to discover creative times and places in which you can squeeze in a few exercises to keep your body feeling relaxed and strong. Make these techniques into a habit—just like eating regular meals! Your stress techniques are important nourishment for your total well-being. Following are a few examples of exercises you've learned earlier in this book and how they can be adapted for everyday use.

AT YOUR DESK:
Seated Twist (p. 179)
Shoulder Rolls (p. 21)
Elbow Touch (p. 22)
Folded Pose (p. 179)
Seated Knee Squeeze (p. 179)
Belly Breath (p. 136)
Complete Breath (p. 137)
Standing Reach (p. 26)
Back Arch (p. 134)
Arm Rolls (p. 23)

IN THE KITCHEN:
Leg Lifts (p. 31)
Arm Rolls (p. 23)
Easy Bend (p. 27)
Alternate Triangle (p. 59)
Standing Reach (p. 26)
Neck Stretch (p. 24)
Lazy Stretch (p. 28)
Easy Balance Twist (p. 55)

WATCHING TELEVISION:
Seated Twist (p. 179)
Seated Knee Squeeze (p. 179)
Folded Pose (p. 179)
Lion (p. 139)
Elbow Touch (p. 22)
Back Arch (p. 134)

IN THE BATHROOM:
Standing Knee Squeeze (p. 32)
Easy Bend (p. 27)
Cat Breath (p. 74)
Tree Pose (p. 64)
Lazy Stretch (p. 28)
Back Arch (p. 134)

ON BUSINESS TRIPS OR VACATION:
Easy Spine Twist (p. 91)
Easy Bridge (p. 104)
Full Bends (p. 28)
Easy Cobra (p. 120)
Baby Pose (p. 53)
Cat Breath (p. 74)
Standing Sun Pose (p. 70)
Half Shoulder Stand (p. 110)

FOOD

No discussion of stress would be complete without talking about what you put *into* your body. A proper diet is essential to fighting the effects of stress. Dr. Hans Selye, the "discoverer" of the stress syndrome, said that most of us experience about fifteen "stress events" per day! Each of these events is accompanied by a drain on the body's reserves of nutrients. If these are not replenished regularly by a varied and balanced diet, the considerable drain can result in illness.

In some ways our bodies haven't changed much over the long evolutionary process. When we are faced with a threat—either real or imaginary—our bodies react instantaneously to ready us for combat (fight) or escape (flight). Selye calls this the alarm stage. It all starts when the brain, through its sensory apparatus, receives and interprets environmental signals to mean that the body is in danger. Messenger hormones carry this "red alert" signal throughout the body, triggering several reactions at once:

1. Blood pressure rises and pulse rate increases, in order to speed the messengers and nutrients along their way.
2. Blood sugar increases (drawn from available proteins first, and then from stores) to provide instant energy if it is required.
3. Vitamin C is mobilized to help fight infection.
4. Calcium and other minerals are drawn from the bones to stimulate muscle tone in case the body has to move quickly.
5. Body functions that are not absolutely necessary to meet this crisis (such as digestion) slow down.
6. Sodium content (and thus water retention) increases in order to prevent dehydration.

All this happens in a split second. Our body is now ready to face the threat (even if the "threat" is only imaginary or is emotional). Doesn't it seem silly that all this happens when someone gives you a sharp word—as if it were a physical attack? Nevertheless, the body does not distinguish between a physical threat or an emotional or mental one; it reacts exactly the same way.

When the "threat" is removed and the alarm is over, the body goes into the second stage—resistance—in which it repairs any damage and continues its various functions. The nutrients that are so necessary during stress must be replenished. Protein, once it has been broken down to form sugar for energy, can't be reused as protein; vitamin C and the excess B vitamins are excreted (the so-called water-soluble vitamins only last for about four hours after having been ingested); and minerals cannot be reinserted into the bones.

"Keep Moving" Routine for Any Time of Day

This routine features exercises you can do at your desk. Cut this page out and post in a prominent place in your office or home!

Regular aerobic exercise is important, too. Run up and down stairs; jog around the block; take a brisk walk to the supply room or to lunch—just keep moving!

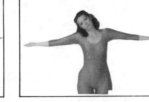

Neck Stretch

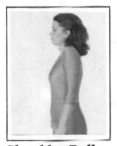
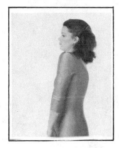
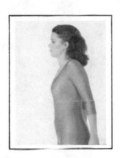

Shoulder Roll

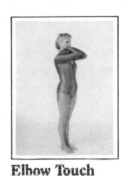

Elbow Touch

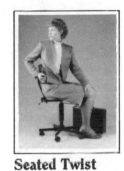

Seated Twist

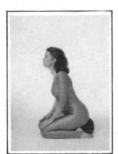

Back Arch

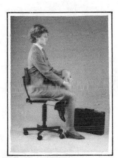

Seated Knee Squeeze

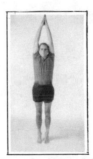

Standing Reach

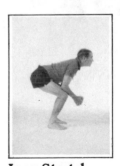

Lazy Stretch

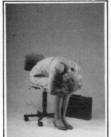

Folded Pose

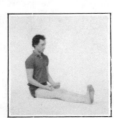

Foot Flaps

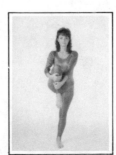

Standing Knee Squeeze

Now it is easy to see the importance of eating correctly in order to meet the constant demands of stress. The essential nutrients must be ingested in sufficient amounts to ensure adequate supplies not only to help out during the stress event but also to do their normal jobs in the body during our almost continuous resistance stage: repair, rebuilding and normal growth and change according to our age, sex, state of health and other factors.

The best way to protect yourself against the depletion of these necessary nutrients is to make the most of each "eating occasion." Ideally, five or six small meals are better than the pattern with which many of us are familiar: minimal breakfast, coffee and sweet midmorning, fast-food lunch, large dinner. If six small meals are not feasible for you (or if you are afraid you won't be able to control the amount of calories taken in at each small meal), the next best thing is to have a good breakfast and lunch, a light dinner, and high-protein, low-calorie snacks between meals. (See nutrition chapter for snack suggestions.) Eat dinner early in the evening and avoid snacking later, so you'll be hungry for breakfast. Eating early also helps burn off some of what you've eaten instead of letting it sit there while your body tries to digest during the night when it needs to be resting. Do you eat more junk foods when you are in a hurry, or often go on fad diets? If so, you may be compounding your stress reactions with poor eating habits. Read the discussion about your nutrition life-style in the chapter on nutrition.

Enemies of a stress-resistant diet are: caffeine, alcohol, excessive sugar, smoking and processed and refined foods. All these wildly manipulate blood sugar levels and/or add empty calories. By substituting more healthy snacks for caffeine and sugar, your body will achieve a more gradual rise in blood sugar, which will be sustained longer. After work, try a yoga "happy hour" instead of alcohol. Besides the obvious physical dangers, alcohol dulls your sensitivity to what is happening in your body and mind—exactly the opposite effect from what is desired in yoga. Smoking reduces the amount of vitamin C in your body, so you may wish to consider keeping a bottle of chewable tablets on your desk to help lick the cigarette habit.

BREATH—YOUR MOST PORTABLE STRESS MANAGEMENT TOOL

Remember when someone said, "Just sit down and take a few deep breaths and you'll feel better"? It usually worked, didn't it? Do you know why?

You may have noticed how your breath changes when you get excited, tense, angry or upset. The reverse also works. You can achieve a change in your mental state by consciously changing your breath. An anxious or disturbed mind (one ready for "fight or flight") creates a vicious cycle of tight breath patterns and frantic thoughts. Knowing how to use yoga breathing exercises can be your best—and most readily available—stress management tool. Breathing exercises can help you recover much more quickly from a stress event by manipulating your state of mind into a more quiet level.

The Belly Breath (see Chapter 5, p. 136) is the best way to change your state of mind instantly. If you sit or stand straight, consciously relax and push out your stomach as you breathe in and squeeze as you breathe out, concentrating on the sound of the breath in the back of your throat, you will break that vicious cycle of stressed mind/stressed breath and notice a difference within a few minutes.

Many people who often have trouble sleeping at night find that doing breathing exercises in bed helps them relax, get their mind off the daily events and get to sleep. Do the Belly Breath, as slowly as possible without straining, and try to concentrate on the sound of the breath alone. The right food can also help. Having a high-carbohydrate dinner and bedtime snack makes your body feel more relaxed and drowsy.

RELAXATION AND MEDITATION

Have you ever felt confused, frustrated or angry after a stressful incident and, later, when you were more relaxed and clearheaded, wondered how you could have reacted so strongly about something so trivial? That shows how your thinking patterns change when you're under stress. It's almost as if the mind reverts to a more primitive, reactive state and judges only in terms of survival. When you're stressed you probably are less able to concentrate and less patient with interruptions, and you may find it difficult to be creative.

Sometimes there are simply so many things crowding into your consciousness at once that your mind becomes jumbled and anxious just because you can't decide what the priorities are. At these times try drawing back from *everything* for a minute or two. Giving your conscious mind a break often allows your uncon-

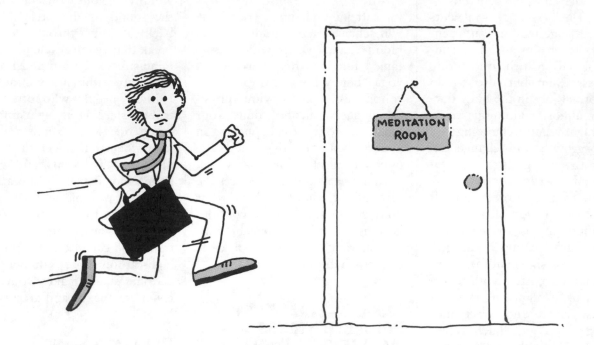

scious to sort things out and let the important things come forward. It's like getting a second opinion on your problems!

Practicing daily relaxation and meditation as part of your yoga routine can help most by giving you a foundation for achieving a more stable and aware outlook. If you work at remembering how it feels, during meditation, to be completely still and relaxed, you can reproduce that feeling whenever you need it or want it during the day. However, you can also benefit from doing a shorter version of the meditation technique.

If you can find a quiet, uninterrupted spot for five or ten minutes (your office, a conference room or even the bathroom), try a short meditation to give yourself this kind of minivacation from responsibilities and problems. When you return you will be refreshed, calmer and ready to tackle the rest of the day with new energy.

If you can, wash your hands and sprinkle water on your face first. Then sit comfortably, hands in your lap, eyes closed. Take a few deep, full breaths, concentrating on the sound as you breathe in and out smoothly and evenly. Then let your breath relax. Consciously relax your face, paying special attention to the tiny muscles around your eyes and the muscles of your jaw. Relax your shoulders, arms and hands, and stomach. Relax your legs and feet; the back of your neck and your head. Feel your whole body go limp, but don't slouch: Keep your back straight. Then, for the next few minutes, try to be silent inside. You'll notice the emotions and problems trying to crowd into your awareness, but try to keep them away. If it helps, imagine a screen or sky filling your whole consciousness. Remember how stillness feels when you are doing your meditation practice at home. Melt into the silence; let it surround you and fill you up. Rest in

it. After a few minutes, start breathing more deeply. Stretch your arms, and imagine yourself filled with renewed energy and strength. Then go back to your work.

Even when you are not particularly stressed, using this technique can help you get a clearer idea of how your mind works. You may be able to find out what upsets or concerns you most—and why. You might even be able to make some decisions about how to spend your energy more wisely.

GO FOR IT!

If you know how to manage it, stress can work to your advantage. With the right attitude and knowledge or appropriate techniques, anything that life puts in front of you can be approached as a challenge instead of an obstacle. Yoga is in your corner!

CHAPTER 11
PHILOSOPHIES FOR LIFE

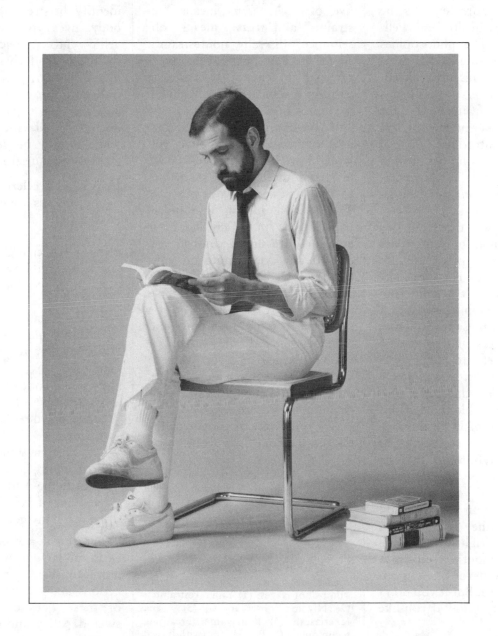

In yoga, experience is everything. The only way to learn something about yoga is to do it. Yoga has no precepts or beliefs that everyone must follow to be a yoga student. You are never expected to believe anything unless it happens to you. However, what most people find as they continue to practice yoga is that certain attitudes about everyday living begin to make more sense as the effects of better health and well-being increase. The philosophies of yoga are not intellectual exercises; rather, they resemble an applied psychology of self that forms a protective framework for growth in yoga practice. This chapter will introduce you to some of the basic concepts of yoga philosophy and the attitudes, values and behaviors that characterize a yogic life-style.

As you read through this chapter, there may be some ideas that you find strange at first, or even unacceptable. This does not mean that you can't benefit from your practices! Don't believe that you *must* adopt these ideas before you can progress. There are no mandatory beliefs. In yoga, ideas and attitudes are expressed solely to enhance the learning experience by removing possible distractions and obstacles to growth. In reading this chapter, try to adopt an attitude of playfulness. Try the concepts on for size. Think about them in terms of your own life, and then make your own decision about whether they fit in or not. Some will fit in right away. Some may fit in six months from now. And some may never fit. It is entirely your choice. But if you don't try it, you won't know if you like it or not.

The following brief overview of yoga philosophy is a gentle way of expanding your ways of thinking about life and especially ways of living as a yoga student.

GUIDELINES FOR INTEGRITY: YAMAS AND NIYAMAS

In the classical yoga system there are ten ethical guidelines called the yamas and niyamas. There are five of each. *Yama* means "restraint," and *niyama* means "observance" (literally, nonrestraint). These are part of the eight stages of yoga practice that were set forth by a scholar named Patanjali a couple of thousand years ago.*

If you had happened to be curious about yoga at that time, you would have been expected to have mastered these ethical guidelines as your first step in yoga practice. The classical idea is that unless your life is in order and your emotions are under control, you can't really concentrate on your mind. Nowadays, the techniques seem to be what is most important. You start with exercises, you may learn some breathing and meditation, and only then, if you've decided that you want to make more changes in your life, do you go on to study these ethical guidelines more seriously.

Are you aware of knowing a little more about how your mind

*There are various opinions about when Patanjali lived, spanning several centuries around the birth of Christ. However, no one doubts his contribution: the organization of all the various schools of yoga that were being practiced in India in his time. His description of what is known as Classical Yoga breaks down the practice into eight "limbs" or stages: (1) Yama (restraints); (2) Niyama (observances); (3) Asana (exercises); (4) Pranayama (breathing techniques); (5) Pratyahara (withdrawal of the mind from the senses); (6) Dharana (concentration); (7) Dhyana (meditation); (8) Samadhi (absorption).

and body work since you started your yoga practice? This practice of observation and self-awareness is central to yoga. Although observation is key in all phases of your technique practice—your exercises, breathing and meditation—this inner-directed observation begins, at some point, to spill over into everyday life. For example, by observation you learn to identify the stress signals that your body gives you before they develop into full-scale problems such as headaches or stomach upset. Similarly, as your concentration improves, you find that you are able to work more productively and efficiently. After a while it may be very natural to start asking questions like these:

How can I accelerate this observation process in my life?

How can I find out more about what I am observing?

How much change do I want in my life, and how will yoga help me bring about the desired changes?

What do I really want out of life, and how much time and effort am I willing to put toward getting it?

How much control do I have over what happens to me?

What is my direction or purpose in life?

What are some things that distract me from my goals, and how can I reduce the distraction?

What kind of behavior best helps me reach my goals?

The *yamas* and *niyamas* are the extra effort yogis make to become more conscious of their motives, actions and feelings so that some of these questions can be answered. Study and practice of the yamas and niyamas help to deepen the experience of self-awareness beyond the level of normal physical consciousness. In this way they work to eliminate any conscious or unconscious impediments to growth.

Let's look at the first and one of the most important of the yamas —nonviolence (ahimsa). Most people do not find it difficult to obey the laws of the land against violence. We have very strict penalties for such behavior and strong moral proscriptions against it. Consider the behavior of children: Their responses are almost totally instinctive or automatic. As they grow up, they have to learn not to hit, not to yell and so on in hurtful ways. Most adults, however, still do these things internally, with a similar emotional disturbance. Our most uncontrollable emotional upsets are those that are so ingrained or reinforced by years of practice that they are automatic.

The yogi, through concentration, awareness and attention, tries to remove these automatic responses as much as possible. Then the yogi takes the idea of nonviolence one step further by refraining from harmfulness through thought or word in addition to action. Think of how many times in a moment of anger you may have thought to yourself, "I hate you! I wish you were dead! I wish you'd get out of my life forever!"—and regretted it afterward, because you didn't really mean it? Yogis believe that thoughts can hurt as well as words or weapons. For a while, that use of violence will echo in the unconscious with all the other unfinished business, but the results of that violence will eventually have to be faced and dealt with.

So the yamas and niyamas are ways of modifying outward life so that it conforms with our inner ideals. This does not mean that yogis are totally unemotional. A common misconception is the image of a serene yogi sitting on top of a mountain in perfect peace. In fact, many yoga students, when they are first trying to practice, receive gentle and not-so-gentle ribbing on the lines of "How come you're upset? I thought you were practicing yoga!" which sometimes can be very hard to counter. However, it is true that a yogi does not get emotionally disturbed as often, because he or she decides not to waste energy on things that are not worth it. As awareness and concentration increase, you will be able to make a decision about your response to a situation instead of the response being automatic. Observance of the yamas and niyamas helps you choose your responses.

We've already discussed the first yama, nonviolence or harmlessness (ahimsa), which is one of the most important ones. This attitude and behavior toward all living creatures is based on the recognition of the underlying unity of all life. And so nonviolence is behind the idea of vegetarianism (see the Nutrition chapter for more information). The yogi goes even further, though, and resolves to let go of those automatic responses of anger or resentment or frustration that don't do him or her any good. Most important, nonviolence includes the concept of harmlessness toward oneself. A yogi who seriously practices nonviolence will work very hard to eliminate any self-destructive actions or omissions from his or her life, such as smoking, skipping meals or failing to fasten the seat belt.

Patanjali offers an unusual and delightful promise with each of the yamas: "Every temptation that [a yogi] overcomes, is tantamount to a force that he makes his own."[*] If nonviolence is practiced perfectly, Patanjali says, this restraint turns itself into a positive force of love. Because of his practice, the yogi gains a realization of the unity of all life and can never be harmed.

Not lying, or truthfulness (satya), is the second yama: Satya includes exaggeration, equivocation and pretense. However, truthfulness is never more important than nonviolence. If a yogi would cause harm by telling the truth, Patanjali says, he or she should be silent instead. The practice of truthfulness also brings about its reward: the development of intuition. Intuition is a mental function all of us have. Normally its access is blocked by emotional turbulence; although now and then you have probably experienced a "flash" of insight that comes from this little-used area of your mind. With the conscious practice of restraining the negative energy that goes into changing or hiding the truth, you can make more opportunities for intuition to come forward. With time, you can gain access to that mental function at will.

The third yama is not-stealing (asteya), sometimes called non-misappropriation. This includes not only not stealing things but also ideas—into taking credit for something you didn't do—and unearned privilege. This also turns into its opposite, the reward of having everything you need.

The fourth—and most misunderstood—yama is celibacy (bramacharya). This is a tough one, because celibacy fits so easily into the ascetic mold that most people associate with yoga. The important thing about celibacy training

*Eliade, Mircea, Patanjali and Yoga, p. 65.

is that it teaches you to become more aware of how much of your reactions are manipulated by the outside world (especially by the media) to stimulate your sexual desire. Sex is, of course, a very motivating force in our lives, the essence of the continuation of all life. But this constant manipulation of our desires takes a great deal of energy. Celibacy practice allows you to rest from this powerful pull for short periods of time so that you can more clearly observe how your mind and emotions work. Celibacy includes mental abstinence as well as physical.

As a clarifying exercise, you may wish to try practicing celibacy for a short period of time. At first, set aside five minutes at the same time every day, during which you try to observe every thought, reaction and perception that crosses your mind and attempt to eliminate those that are stimulated by an automatic sexual response. If you like, you can extend the time to an hour each week. You may even want to try one full day each week. You may find that not only do you have more (and more focused) energy for your life, but also that your love relationships become more tender and deeper as new channels of communication open.

Celibacy can also be used as a protection against destructive sexual behavior during periods of loss or depression. After a separation, divorce or broken love affair, a person sometimes reaches for the temporary closeness of casual sex to assuage terrible loneliness. During these times a short commitment to celibacy can protect a person from the emotional and physical hazards of promiscuity.

The fifth yama is *nonpossessiveness (aparigraha)*, the practice of detachment. This is a tricky concept to understand, because not only do you have to decide what you wish to become detached from, but also you must take care that you are not simply withdrawing from difficult or unwanted responsibilities as an escape and calling it detachment.

There are some things from which it is impossible to be detached and still remain able to attain your goals. Breath, for example, consciousness and the desire to live are absolutely necessary. These are obvious, you may think. But a yogi learns to assume nothing and to take nothing for granted in the search for self-knowledge.

Detachment also has to do with the balance of responsibility and withdrawal. For most people, attention and awareness are almost completely externally directed—in reaction to their relationships and social life, their job, their community and the like. In yoga, you begin to transfer some of that attention and awareness inside, as you start learning more about yourself and how your mind, body, emotions and unconscious work. However, no real yoga teacher will tell you that you must withdraw completely and run away to the mountains in order to achieve anything. Yoga teaches that you must learn to bring your new knowledge about your inner self into balance and harmony with your outer self.

"Yoga is skill in action," says the Bhagavad Gita (see box, p. 192). In yoga, you must bring order and fulfillment and meaning to every single detail of your life. So the ties of close relationships, the pull of talents and career goals—these are things a human being must continue to acknowledge in order to become fully human.

A yogi who attempts to practice detachment observes an interesting phenomenon: his or her desires gradually decrease! As the flurry of automatic responses to advertising or stress or boredom diminishes, the drive to acquire also subsides. Then goals can become more clearly defined.

Now we move to the *niyamas*, or "observances." These are qualities that you practice to protect and strengthen yourself, build your concentration and reinforce your desire to keep learning.

Purity (saucha) is the first niyama—the maintenance and transformation of the vehicle through which we strive for our goals. The body is "tuned up" through the right food, drink, exercise, general health maintenance, rest, cleanliness, relief from stress and so on. The mind is purified through observation and meditation—the removal of disturbances through present-moment quietness.

Contentment (santosh) is the second niyama. This is an idea of equilibrium, of being happy with where you are, but having a clear idea of where you are going. Contentment does not mean stagnation, resting on your laurels or coasting along with no direction. Contentment has to do with "process" as well as "goal." When you are doing the Sun Pose, for example, and you are concentrating mentally on the vision of yourself performing the perfect pose, you will add beauty to the exercise if you also keep your awareness on the *process* of each movement toward the goal. In each step of an exercise, and especially during the transitions between exercises, you should try to maintain the present-moment awareness, proper breathing and muscle use, so that the experience of each movement is as fulfilling as the completed pose.

The third niyama is *discipline* or austerity *(tapas)*. Both these words unfortunately have negative connotations of pain and hardship. But in yoga, and in many aspects of life, discipline means self-control—a valued quality without which it is nearly impossible to reach worthwhile goals. The guidelines that you adopt for the purpose of nurturing your individual growth, whether they be exercise, nutritional support, meditation, ethical behavior or many other positive actions, are the foundation for the development of the concentration, willpower and energy needed to attain your goals.

Study (svadhyaya) is the fourth niyama: reading, reflection, trying to apply the concepts to life. Study creates a deliberate thought and action based on what you've learned and what you've read, and reduces the likelihood that you will be confused or misled by your experiences.

The fifth niyama is *remembrance (ishwara-pranidhana)*. This is an acknowledgment or a recognition of the nondying part of yourself and its manifestation in all life. Whatever name you give to it—God or the Self or the Oversoul or whatever—the essential idea is one of unity with that. A remembrance of this is necessary in order to collaborate with the yogi's desire for unity and integration. This quality also fills your life with beauty and delight as you learn to appreciate all the myriad variations of life in the world.

The way to start practicing the yamas and niyamas is to first observe how they may already be part of your daily life. Then pick one to concentrate on for a period of time—perhaps a week, a month or even a year. Try to keep track of all the little ways that that principle asserts itself in your everyday affairs. You may be surprised at how often the issue that you've chosen comes up in daily life! Make a conscious effort to change your actions and reactions to reflect the principle that you are trying to put into practice.

Patanjali recommends the implantation of the opposite thought; for example, when a violent thought comes up, it should be replaced by a loving thought. This has to do with the power of mental focus. The mind is more powerful than most of us think. There is an old Buddhist saying: As a man thinks, so he becomes. The more you *think* about and *envision* yourself becoming a certain way, the more likely you are to *become* that way. The yamas and niyamas open new mental channels and create conscious behavior patterns to replace old, unconscious habits. If you would like to find out more about them, see The Suggested Reading List.

Practice of the yamas and niyamas means that the yogi has taken responsibility for his or her own life. This idea of responsibility can be extended even further, by examining the idea of *karma* and reincarnation.

ACCEPTING RESPONSIBILITY FOR LIFE: KARMA AND REINCARNATION

Reincarnation is the concept of living not only one life but many lives. In this way of thinking, the soul, spirit or self—whatever you choose to call the undying part of you—at the body's death simply moves on to a new body, with its new agendas, new problems to figure out, new relationships, new formations or manifestations of talents. But the new identity is based upon the old one. In other words, the strengths and weaknesses that have been developed over the course of a lifetime will carry over into the next. This is one way to explain child prodigies such as Mozart, who was composing and playing masterpieces at the age of four. A yogi would say that in a previous life Mozart was so involved in music that the talent carried over urgently and strongly into the next life.

Reincarnation would not make much sense without looking at the idea of *karma*. The word in Sanskrit means literally "action." Karma is the idea that your actions, your thoughts and your desires—literally every impulse that comes from you—all have appropriate consequences. These consequences may occur immediately (such as getting a ticket for parking illegally) or perhaps next year, or even, perhaps, in another life. This means that we are inevitably and ultimately responsible for our actions, our thoughts, and our desires, and for the consequences of those actions. It's sort of like Newton's law: For every action there is an equal and opposite reaction.

Many people think of karma in the same terms as fate, or destiny, which has been predetermined by some outside agency or force. But karma is both initiated and perpetuated only by oneself—by all of one's thoughts, desires and actions that weave the results of our life's actions into a complicated fabric.* When the cloth is already

*There is a marvelous story about a miserly merchant in old Baghdad who resists change, which illustrates this concept perfectly: "Abu Kasems' Slippers," told in Heinrich Zimmer's *The King and the Corpse* (see Bibliography).

woven so intricately, it becomes like an old friend. It is composed of all the pieces of our social and individual personalities, painstakingly fitted and joined into a conscious and unconscious picture of who and what we are. When our growth demands that we dismantle that tapestry, it is often very difficult to do so because it has been with us for so long.

So karma says that life is constantly changing, and we are constantly discovering new experiences, new puzzles about life and new ways of dealing with them. Karma says that you have to work out these problems or you will be presented with them repeatedly until the lesson is learned. Have you ever known somebody who encounters the same kind of situation in love or career over and over again, making the same mistake each time? This is the kind of repeated experience that may be trying to tell that person something about himself or herself—that some kind of change in response is needed before the individual can go forward with life.

This is the real lesson of karma. We are responsible for our own growth. If our lives do not go as planned, we can't blame it on the church, we can't blame it on our parents or society or anything or anybody else. *We* must decide how we shall live in the world. One of the jewels of yoga is that it shows us how to learn to become the masters of our own lives, instead of settling for being servants of circumstance. The idea in yoga is to become aware of the tendencies and characteristics that lie in the subconscious impelling us to react in certain ways, so they can be changed for the better. It's an opportunity for finding out more about ourselves—our motives, goals, fears, strengths, weaknesses, likes, dislikes, habits, and

so on. That kind of awareness and control gives an irreplaceable happiness, because you are then not bound by habits or characteristics you don't like. You become truly free to choose how you want to be. You aren't stuck with a characteristic that does you no good! For example, if you have a bad temper, you can learn to change that reaction to a more appropriate and less destructive one.

Can you think of something in your own life that is unfinished business? A scenario that seems to happen again and again; and to which you always react in the same way? Do you look back and wonder why it is that you can never learn?

What is there about your everyday behavior that you think you might like to change? Take a moment to write down some of these things. Yoga practice offers a way of building the skills, the will, the concentration and the steadiness to be able to tackle these changes effectively, so that your life can be as expansive and beautiful and fulfilling as you would like it to be.

PERCEPTION AND REALITY: MAYA

What are the types of thoughts and feelings that most interfere with your meditation? Make a list. You might include things like a recent argument or an especially pleasant experience; other stressors, personal situations; your shopping list, your "to do" list at work; a major decision that you've been considering. Most of these distractions have to do with either past or future, don't they? So by attempting to be more present-minded in meditation, you are also strengthening your ability

to dwell less on these distractions at other times. Your breathing and exercises, moreover, help develop control by increasing your concentration and teaching you to focus on one thing at a time.

In your everyday life you can make that process even more conscious by thinking about what really matters to you. What do you really, really, really want in your life? And the second most important question is: how much time, effort, thought and concentration do you put into getting or achieving it? This is where you can use the strength of discipline to support your goals. In addition, a clearer perception can smooth your way as you try to reach them. The concept of *maya* has to do with this idea of perception.

Let's talk about perception for a moment. Did you eat dinner yesterday? How do you know that? Memory, of course. But memory can be deceiving, as everybody knows. Witnesses can have entirely different stories about what happened in an accident, based on their point of view. It seems that we live most of our lives on assumptions because of the way our brains work.

Scientists tell us that the brain is presented constantly with a myriad of sensory input from our eyes, ears, fingers, skin and so on. However, there is a filtering process in our minds that allows us to remember only a portion of those perceptions—that portion the mind decides is important. Indeed, if we had to remember *all* of our perceptions we would be overwhelmed, because there would be so many. So there has to be some kind of filter. That filter is constructed, over the course of our lives, by our perspective on the world. Every single individual has a different world and sees things in a slightly different way. Even if you grow up in the same house as someone else, your memories are different, the things that you consider important are different and, consciously or unconsciously, you make decisions about what to remember and what not to remember. When you think about it, it is really a miracle that we are able to communicate at all!

Maya is the Indian way of describing the confusing realities of the world. Maya is called the world dream, which continually plunges us into our unconscious by confronting us with the paradox of opposites, as represented by our varying perceptions. We *are and are not* what we seem to be; the world *is and is not* what it seems to us; what we experience *is and is not* real. We are both tied to the earth and transcendent. Through yoga we wake up from the dream by becoming more conscious, more aware and more discriminating.*

Since perception is always a filtering process, how do we decide

Vishnu's Maya, a short film, tells a delightful story about maya from Indian mythology. See Bibliography.

what is really real for us? In meditation you start out by withdrawing your attention from the senses, by completely relaxing your body and moving away from the physical consciousness. As your awareness inside increases, you begin to get a much clearer, finer and more subtle picture of yourself—who and what you really are. So the faulty perceptions of our physical consciousness, which are dictated by our personal filters, lose their importance and effect on our state of mind. The constant effort in meditation to maintain the present moment is a step toward discrimination, a step toward not getting distracted from our real goals.

THE ADVENTURE OF SELF-DISCOVERY: MYTHOLOGY AND CHANGE

You may be thinking that this discussion about goals and ways of achieving them reminds you of an adventure story. The search for the self truly is a quest, because it requires us to seek out new experiences and observations, and to explore the complicated world of

our unconscious. Stories, legends, dreams and myths are ways of practicing that journey by becoming familiar with what kinds of experience we are likely to meet up with. These ancient stories provide timeless symbols to guide us in our conscious lives.

There are many different levels of consciousness. Most of us live primarily in the outer, because it is familiar and comfortable, habitual and undemanding. Yoga starts to expose you to the inner levels. First, with the gradual quieting of the mind in meditation, you learn to pass by surface emotional turbulence and to open up to what lies beneath. Then, as your concentration and observation skills improve, you begin to notice more and more about how your mind works and what your personality is composed of, not only in meditation but also in everyday affairs. You begin to experience the myriad possibilities within your grasp that will allow you to become the kind of person you most want to be.

If you could put the essence of yoga into one word, that word would be *transformation*. Yoga enables you to transform yourself into a thinking, thoughtful, creative, sensitive, responsible and aware human being. Yoga is a journey toward maturation of consciousness, and mythology is one way to facilitate that process.

The study of mythology can help make our life's adventure more enjoyable and understandable. The stories and legends of mythologies all over the world tell in symbols the never-ending story of the psychological process of self-discovery. As you read, put yourself in the place of the hero or heroine. You will find, in those stories of heroic feats, long odysseys and overcoming obstacles, many similarities to your own

---

The unconscious sends all sorts of vapors, odd beings, terrors, and deluding images up into the mind—whether in dream, broad daylight, or insanity; for the human kingdom, beneath the floor of the comparatively neat little dwelling that we call our conscious mind goes down into unsuspected Aladdin caves. There not only jewels but dangerous jinn abide: the inconvenient or resisted psychological powers that we have not thought or dared to integrate into our lives. And they may remain unsuspected. Or, on the other hand, some chance word, the smell of a landscape, the taste of a cup of tea, or the glance of an eye may touch a magic spring, and then dangerous messengers begin to appear in the brain. These are dangerous because they threaten the fabric of the security into which we have built ourselves and our family. But they are fiendishly fascinating too, for they carry keys that open the whole realm of the desired and feared adventure of the discovery of the self." (Joseph Campbell, *The Hero With a Thousand Faces*.)

Often called "the yogi's handbook," the Bhagavad Gita is a small section of a much longer epic called the Mahabharata. The Gita is a conversation in the middle of a battlefield, at dawn just before the war begins, between Arjuna, a magnificent warrior who is fighting for his rightful kingdom, and Krishna, his charioteer and spiritual advisor. Arjuna sees in both armies his friends, relatives, teachers and neighbors, and loses his will to fight. In the eighteen chapters of the Gita, Krishna explains the many kinds of yoga to Arjuna, saying to him that he must stand up and fight, to fulfill his life's purpose with a conscious attitude and determination, with the equanimity and awareness of yoga. This story is used to illustrate the formidable task that we face when we finally confront the familiar faces of our unconscious fears and delights, useless and useful habits, weaknesses and strengths, and find the skills and courage we need to do battle with those parts of our personality that we must change in order to proceed with life. One of our favorite quotes from the Gita:

"A man should lift himself up by his own efforts. He should never pull himself down. For he is his own best friend, and he is his own worst enemy. For him who has conquered his body and mind, his own mind is his true friend. But for him who has no hold on his body and mind, his own mind will be his worst enemy."

Chapter 2, verses 5–6

evolving adventure to find yourself.

Change: It is a tantalizing but fearful prospect. It holds the hope and promise of becoming closer to your ideal, and the insecurity of letting go of what is most familiar. On the adventure of yoga you start out with a dream of how you could be, like a guiding light in the distance. As you get ready for the journey, making the decision to change, the unconscious resists at first, because it is more comfortable with the status quo.

In yoga you have to have a tremendous courage for change. Do you know the story, told by one of the early Greek philosophers, about the man who had spent his whole life in a cave? One day someone came and led him out into the sunlight, but he was so frightened and bewildered that he ran as fast as he could back into the familiar darkness of his cave. Change is always a risk, and we often cling to pain or hurt or darkness because, although it isn't pleasant, at least it is familiar, and the risk of change means risking more hurt. Not only that, but unfamiliar hurt. There is a line in the Bhagavad Gita (see box) that says, "Like poison in the beginning but like nectar in the end." Change does not always mean pain, but whatever adjustment is required, the result is always worth it. It is always much brighter and better than you have ever imagined. The unknown thing that you are afraid of is the very thing that will lead you to freedom. It is the cocoon of the earthbound caterpillar, which eventually frees him to become the gorgeous butterfly that rides on the wind.

It is a strange paradox that most of us, if asked, would profess to a belief in free will—that we are not locked in to a preset fate or destiny. Yet most of us act

as if this were true, by accepting without question things like illness, depression, family conflict, personal limitations, alcohol or drug abuse, fears, nonfulfillment in religion and many others. We are a bundle of acceptance contracts, signed on the dotted line without any fuss. Acceptance of fear and disunity within our own self is the biggest obstacle to the achievement of a fully integrated personality. We can stop our growth by acceptance of apparent limitations. Yoga provides the impetus to celebrate our self in our freedom to be exactly who and what we want to be. The beauty of yoga is that we are *able* to change. From a yogi's viewpoint, the real tragedy in life would be to be stuck as you are, unable to make a positive change for growth.

By exploring your unconscious, you will begin to recognize the possibilities of your own life. You will discover strengths you didn't know you had and will be able to modify your weaknesses so they don't hold you back. You'll be able to recognize which of your habits and reactions are simply broken records endlessly replaying the stucknesses of many years, and change the ones that no longer fit how you want to be. As the hero in your own adventure, you can say to yourself: "*I* am here. This is *my* experience. How do *I* feel about it and what am *I* going to do? I am not going to react in these preprogrammed ways but instead I am going to react the way I need to."

Perhaps you can see now how these concepts fit together. Study and observance of the *yamas and niyamas* offer you guidelines for your behavior and practices that will keep you from being distracted from your objectives.

Through the idea of *karma,* you learn to accept responsibility for your life and recognize that you have the power to change. The concept of *maya* teaches that each person's view of reality is different, and that you must try to clarify what you want your life to be based on the truest perceptions and realizations you can find. *Mythology* gives you examples, in symbols familiar to your unconscious, of the psychological tasks you must accomplish in order to achieve the growth and development you have decided you want.

Think of it as self-realization on the installment plan! If you approach each day with its special messages and challenges, you will begin to enjoy the experience of the present moment not just in meditation but in everyday life. With yoga in your life you will never be bored, because you will have the happiness of knowing that you are on your way to achieving the goals you have set for yourself, whatever they may be. The treasures that wait for you along the way are the richness of experience, the warmth of friendship and love, the excitement of challenge and the wonder of discovery.

GLOSSARY

Agni Kriya—an advanced breathing exercise, introduced in Course Three, involving manipulation of the diaphragm while the breath is held out.

Ahimsa—"non-violence," one of the five *yamas,* or restraints.

Ajna Chakra—a state of consciousness in which intuitive wisdom becomes more accessible; represented in the body by the spot between the eyebrows.

Aparigraha— "nonpossessiveness," one of the five *yamas.*

Asan, or Asana—a position, posture, or movement in yoga exercise.

Asan Point—in practicing asans, the point at which the body is maintained in a relaxed and attentive hold: breath relaxed, mind steady, no unnecessary muscles tensed.

Asteya—"Not stealing," one of the five *yamas.*

Bandha—a lock, or a tightening, of particular muscle groups.

Bee Breath (Brahmari Breath)—a breathing technique introduced in Course Two in which fingers close off sensory input organs and the breath is exhaled as long as possible with a "zzz" sound.

Belly Breath—the introductory breath exercise which teaches use of the diaphragm through emphasis in movement of the lower abdomen.

Brahmacharya—"celibacy," one of the five *yamas.*

Brahmari Breath—*See* Bee Breath.

Complete Breath—a breath exercise encompassing three stages: belly expansion, rib expansion sideways, and chest expansion; the sequence is reversed in exhalation. Inhalation and exhalation are of even lengths.

Dharana— "concentration," the sixth step or "limb" in Patanjali's system of classical yoga.

Dhyana—"meditation," the seventh step in the eight "limbs" of Patanjali's system of classical yoga.

Easy Breath—a breath pattern that is completely nonmanipulated, used in holding positions in asans.

Ekagrata—the ability to focus the mind voluntarily on an object without interruption for extended periods of time.

Hinduism—the major religion of India.

Humming Breath—a breath exercise that involves a short inhalation and long exhalation while making a humming sound.

Ishwara - Pranidhana — "remembrance," one of the five *niyamas,* or observances.

Kapalabhati—an advanced breathing exercise introduced in Course Two involving a period of short "bellows" breaths followed by a deep exhalation, inhalation and an extended, silent exhalation.

Karma—the idea that every action, thought, or desire has an equal and opposite reaction, or appropriate result.

Kashmir Shaivism—a little-known branch of yoga philosophy and practice that emphasizes the basic unity of oneself and the world.

Kinesthetic Sense—the awareness of where your body is in space.

Mantram—a particular sound that is used to bring about a specific result in consciousness.

Maya—the notion that what one perceives as the real world is actually more like a dream because of the many conflicting realities and perceptions caused by differing points of view and understanding.

Meditation—a state of complete silence and inactivity within the conscious mind.

Metabolism—the systems of the body involved in the production and utilization of energy.

Mulabhanda—a lock, or tightening, of the rectal muscles.

Neti—a nasal cleansing technique using warm saltwater.

Niyamas—five "observances" outlined in Patanjali's *Yoga Sutras.*

Om—the mantram used to represent the silence and stillness of meditation.

Patanjali—a scholar of about the sixth century who collected and organized all the systems of yoga in India in his time into a treatise called the *Yoga Sutras,* which describe all the techniques and aims of yoga.

Pranayama—the breathing techniques of yoga.

Pratyahara—"the withdrawal of the mind from the senses," an essential first step in meditation; step five in Patanjali's eight "limbs."

Reincarnation—the notion that the soul or spirit does not die when the body dies but goes on to enter a new body and to continue its development.

Samadhi— "absorption," the eighth step in Patanjali's eight "limbs" of classical yoga.

Santosha—"contentment," one of the five *niyamas*.

Satya—"truth," one of the five *yamas*.

Sauca—"purity," one of the five *niyamas*.

Svadyaya—"study," one of the five *niyamas*.

Tapas—"discipline," one of the five *niyamas*.

Tidal Volume—the amount of air that is moved in and out of the lungs when in a resting state.

Vital Capacity—the total amount of air that can be inhaled.

Yamas—the five "restraints" of Patanjali's system of classical yoga.

Yoga—from the Sanskrit *yug* meaning to join together or to yoke. A set of various techniques for harmony of mind and body within the individual, and harmony between the individual self and the universal self.

Yogi—strictly speaking, one who has attained yoga, or union, but used commonly to refer to anyone who practices yoga techniques on a committed basis.

YOGA TECHNIQUES
CLASSIFIED BY TYPE

Abdomen
Pelvic Twist
All Sit-ups
Cobra V-raise
Ankle Stretch
Alternate Toe Touch
Seated Sun Pose
Sun Balance
Plow Breath
Back Strengtheners
Boat

Ankles
Baby Pose
Easy Balance
Easy Balance Twist
Hero Variation
Standing Reach
Ankle Stretch
Massage
Foot Flaps
Hero Pose

Back, Lower
Knee Squeeze
Easy Bridge
Full Bend
Hip Rock
Side Triangle
Alternate Triangle
Twisting Triangle
Dancer Pose
Pigeon Pose
Roll
Pelvic Twist
Walk
Bow
Hero Variation
Plank
Bow Variation
Camel
Spine Twist
Diamond
Floor Stretch
Sun Salutation

Alternate Sit-up
Cat Breath
Cat Variation
Hero Pose
Boat
Fish
Back Strengtheners
Alternate Toe Touch
Standing Knee Squeeze
Cobra
T Pose
Cobra V-raise
Hands and Knees Stretch
Dancer
Airplane

Back, Upper, and Neck
Arm Roll
Standing Reach
Elbow Twist
Sun Salutation
Easy Bend
Extended Sun Pose
Twisting Triangle
Neck Stretch
Plow
Extended Hero
Side Stretch
Cobra V-raise
Floor Stretch
Plank
Back Strengtheners
Spine Twist
Easy Cobra
Easy Sit Up
Neck Curl
Arm & Leg Balance
Cat Variation
Airplane Series
Fish

Balance
Tree
Standing Reach
Leg Lifts

Complete Leg Lift
Standing Knee Squeeze
Easy Balance and Twist
Dancer Pose
T Pose
Knee Bends

Breathing
Standing Reach
Lazy Stretch
Full Bend
Hands and Knees Stretch
Plow Breath
Easy Balance
Easy Balance Twist
Windmill
Tree Pose
Extended Sun
Extended Hero
Standing Sun Pose
Airplane
Camel
Pigeon
Spine Twist
Shoulder Stand
Floor Stretch
Sun Salutation
Fish Pose

To Relieve Depression
Twisting Triangle
Windmill
Dancer Pose
Lion
Laughasan
Knee Squeeze
Breathing Techniques

Digestion
Standing Knee Squeeze
Knee Squeeze
Baby Pose
Folded Pose
Seated Knee Squeeze
Hip Rock

Spine Twist
Standing Sun Pose
Cat Breath
Plow
Hero Variation
Seated Sun
Walk
Big Sit-up
Shoulder Stand
Boat
Back Strengtheners
Bow
Full Triangle
Twisting Triangle
Plow Breath
Cobra

Eyesight
Spine Twist
Fish Pose
Easy Bridge
Shoulder Stand

Hips and Thighs
Windmill
All Triangles
Complete Leg Lift
Hip Rock and Rotation
T Pose
T Pose Knee Bends
Dancer
Alternate Sit-up
Alternate Toe Touch
Arm and Leg Balance
Bow Variation
Hands and Knees Stretch
Hero Pose
Thigh Stretch
Baby Pose
Stretching Dog
Limber Hips
Big Sit-up

Pigeon
Hero Variation
Sun Balance
Camel
Diamond
Fish
Sun Salutation

Knees
Massage
Knee Bends
Hands and Knees Stretch
Baby Pose
Hero Pose
Camel
Hero Variation
Limber Hips

Legs
Triangles
Sun Poses
Standing Knee Squeeze
Stretching Dog
Leg Lifts
Stretching Dog
Hip Rock
Cobra V-raise
Thigh Stretch
Foot Flap
Lazy Stretch
Full Bend
V-raise, one bent leg
Foot Hold, straighten leg
Stork Stretch

Posture
Elbow Touch
Extended Hero
Sun Pose Variation
Shoulder Roll
Full Bend
Arm and Leg Balance
Plow

Reduce body fat, especially waist
Pelvic Twist
Walk
Alternate Toe Touch
Complete Leg Lift
Alternate Triangle
Cobra V-raise
Hero Variation
Knee Squeeze
Plow

Reproductive System
Diamond
Shoulder Stand
Cobra
Leg Lifts
Baby Pose
Cobra V-raise
Hero Variation
Thigh Stretch
Pigeon Pose
Seated Sun Pose

Shoulders
Shoulder Roll
Elbow Touch
Arm Roll
Stretching Dog
Bow Variation
Plank
Airplane Series
Alternate Sit-up
Extended Hero

Spinal Limberness
Elbow Twist
Spine Twists
Pelvic Twist
Twisting Triangle
Seated Twist

BIBLIOGRAPHY: SOURCES FOR FURTHER STUDY

1. How to Get the Most Out of Yoga

Christensen, Alice. *Yoga, Science and Medicine.* Cleveland, Ohio: The Light of Yoga Society (American Yoga Association), 1975.

Funderburk, R. K. *Science Studies Yoga.* Glenview, Ill.: Himalayan Publications, 1977.

Stiles, Mukunda (Tom). *The Physiology, Psychology, and Philosophy of Yoga: A Bibliography.* San Francisco, Calif.: California Yoga Teachers Association, 1976.

4. Exercise (Asans)

Iyengar, B.K.S. *Light on Yoga.* New York, N.Y.: Schocken Books, 1965.

Swatmarama, Swami. *The Yoga of Light: Hatha Yoga Pradipika.* Commentary by Hans-Ulrich Rieker. New York, N.Y.: Herder and Herder, 1971.

5. Breathing (Pranayama)

Funderburk, R. K. *Science Studies Yoga.* Glenview, Ill.: Himalayan Publications, 1977.

Iyengar, B.K.S. *Light on Pranayama.* New York, N.Y.: Crossroad Publishing Co., 1981.

Sivananda, Swami. *The Science of Pranayama.* Himalayas, India: Divine Life Society, 1978 (dist. in U.S. by Orient Book Distributors, Livingston, N.J.)

6. Relaxation and Meditation

Aurobindo, Shri. *Letters on Yoga,* Volume II. Pondicherry, India: Shri Aurobindo Ashram Publications, 1971.

Christensen, Alice. *Meditation.* Cleveland, Ohio: American Yoga Assoc., 1986.

Jarrell, Howard R. *International Meditation Bibliography.* Metuchen, N.J.: Scarecrow Press, 1985.

7. Yoga and Nutrition

Bland, Dr. Jeffrey. *Nutraerobics.* San Francisco, Calif.: Harper and Row, 1983.

Brody, Jane. *Jane Brody's Nutrition Book.* New York, N.Y.: W. W. Norton & Co., 1981.

———. *The Good Food Book.* New York, N.Y.: Norton, 1985.

Davis, Adelle. *Let's Stay Healthy, A Guide to Lifelong Nutrition.* New York, N.Y.: New American Library, 1983.

Hartbarger, Janie C., and Hartbarger, Neil J. *Eating for the Eighties: A Complete Guide to Vegetarian Nutrition.* Philadelphia, Pa.: The Saunders Press, 1981.

Lappé, Frances M. *Diet for a Small Planet* (revised ed.). New York, N.Y.: Ballantine Books, 1982.

Mindell, Earl. *Vitamin Bible* (revised ed.). New York, N.Y.: Warner Books, 1985.

Null, Gary. *The New Vegetarian Cookbook.* New York, N.Y.: Macmillan Publishing Co., 1980.

Sussman, Vic. S. *The Vegetarian Alternative.* Emmaus, Pa.: Rodale Press, 1978.

PERIODICALS

American Health. American Health Partners, New York, N.Y.

Nutrition Action. Center for Science in the Public Interest, Washington, D.C.

Tufts University Diet and Nutrition Letter. Tufts University Diet and Nutrition Letter, New York, N.Y.

8. Yoga During Pregnancy

Davis, Adelle. *Let's Have Healthy Children.* New York, N.Y.: Harcourt, Brace, Jovanovich, 1972.

Hess, Mary Abbott. *Pickles and Ice Cream: The Complete Guide to Nutrition During Pregnancy.* New York, N.Y.: McGraw-Hill, 1982.

9. Yoga and Sports

Anderson, Bob. *Stretching.* Bolinas, Calif.: Shelter Publications, Inc., 1980.

Couch, Jean and Weaver, Nell. *Runner's World Yoga Book.* Mountain View, Calif.: Runner's World Publications, Inc., 1979.

Elliott, Richard. *The Competitive Edge.* Englewood Cliffs, N.J.: Prentice Hall, 1984.

Mayo, DeBarra. *Yoga, Book II.* Mountain View, Calif.: Runner's World Publ., 1983.

10. Yoga for Stress Management

Ardell, Donald B. *14 Days to a Wellness Lifestyle.* Mill Valley,

Calif.: Whatever Publishing Co., 1982.

Davis, Adelle. *Let's Get Well* (chapter on stress). New York, N.Y.: Harcourt, Brace, and World, 1965.

Selye, Hans. *The Stress of Life* (revised ed.). New York, N.Y.: McGraw-Hill Book Co., 1976.

Tubesing, Donald A. *Kicking Your Stress Habits*. Duluth, Minn.: Whole Person Associates, 1982.

Winston, Stephanie. *Getting Organized*. New York, N.Y.: Warner Books, 1978.

11. Philosophies for Life

Aurobindo, Shri. *Letters on Yoga,* Volume I. Pondicherry, India: Shri Aurobindo Ashram Publications, 1971.

Ball, Thomas. *Vishnu's Maya.* (30-minute film). New York, N.Y.: Phoenix Films, 1975.

Campbell, Joseph. *The Hero With a Thousand Faces.* Princeton, N.J.: Princeton University Press, 1949.

————. *The Masks of God.* New York, N.Y.: Viking Press, 1962.

————. *The Mythic Image.* Princeton, N.J.: Princeton University Press, 1974.

Christensen, Alice. *The Light of Yoga.* Cleveland, Ohio: The American Yoga Association, 1976.

————. *The Joy of Celibacy.* Cleveland, Ohio: The American Yoga Association, 1976.

————. *Reflections of Love.* Cleveland, Ohio: The American Yoga Association, 1982.

Danielou, Alain. *Yoga, the Method of Reintegration.* New York, N.Y.: University Books, 1955.

Eliade, Mircea. *Patanjali and Yoga.* New York, N.Y.: Schocken Books, 1975.

————. *Yoga: Immortality and Freedom.* Princeton, N.J.: Princeton University Press, 1958.

Jarrell, Howard R. *International Yoga Bibliography.* Metuchen, N.J.: Scarecrow Press, 1981.

Kulkarni, V. G., trans. *The Bhagavad Gita.* Cleveland, Ohio: Laxmi Enterprises, 1978.

Sivananda, Swami, trans. *The Bhagavad Gita.* Sivanandanagar, India: The Divine Life Society, 1969.

Taimni, I. K. *The Science of Yoga.* Wheaton, Ill.: Theosophical Publishing House, 1961.

Venkatesananda, Swami. *Enlightened Living.* (Interpretation and commentary on Patanjali's Yoga Sutra.) New Delhi, India: Motilal Banarsidass, 1975.

Vivekananda, Swami. *Raja Yoga.* New York, N.Y.: Ramakrishna/Vivekananda Center, 1982.

Yogananda, Paramhansa. *Autobiography of a Yogi.* Los Angeles, Calif.: Self-Realization Fellowship, 1977.

Zimmer, Heinrich. *The King and the Corpse: Tales of the Soul's Conquest of Evil.* Princeton, N.J.: Princeton University Press, 1957.

————. *Myths and Symbols in Indian Art and Civilization.* Princeton, N.J.: Princeton University Press, 1946.

INDEX

ABOUT THE AUTHOR

Alice Christensen is the Executive Director of the American Yoga Association, which has offices in Cleveland, Ohio, and Sarasota, Florida. She began her education in Classical Yoga with Swami Sivananda in Rishkesh, India, in 1952, and continues advanced yoga studies in India several months a year to this day. In 1965 she became the first woman to lecture on Yoga and Vedantic Philosophy at New Delhi University in India, and in 1981 she received a Letter of Commendation from the Ohio House of Representatives for her work with the community. Currently, Ms. Christensen divides her time between Cleveland and Sarasota.

The American Yoga Association has two locations in the United States:

P.O. Box 18487   513 S. Orange Avenue
Cleveland, Ohio 44118   Sarasota, Florida 33577